Healthcare
Reflections, Insights, and Lessons

ProActive/ReActive

Steven J Sobak

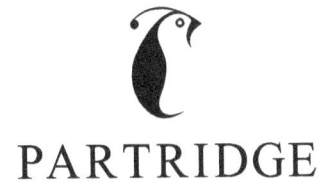

PARTRIDGE

Copyright © 2019 by Steven J Sobak.

Library of Congress Control Number: 2019913483
ISBN: Hardcover 978-1-5437-5394-3
Softcover 978-1-5437-5392-9
eBook 978-1-5437-5393-6

All rights reserved. No part of this book may be used or reproduced by any means, graphic, electronic, or mechanical, including photocopying, recording, taping or by any information storage retrieval system without the written permission of the author except in the case of brief quotations embodied in critical articles and reviews.

Because of the dynamic nature of the Internet, any web addresses or links contained in this book may have changed since publication and may no longer be valid. The views expressed in this work are solely those of the author and do not necessarily reflect the views of the publisher, and the publisher hereby disclaims any responsibility for them.

Print information available on the last page.

To order additional copies of this book, contact
Toll Free 800 101 2657 (Singapore)
Toll Free 1 800 81 7340 (Malaysia)
orders.singapore@partridgepublishing.com

www.partridgepublishing.com/singapore

"A good practical textbook of healthcare management should not only lay down the standard principles of management, but also seek to impart general knowledge of real-life experiences across the contexts of health care settings. Steve Sobak has done this in his publication, which gives rich personal insights that goes beyond many common concepts with the thoughtful considerations of the practitioner. He presents not just practical issues but gives concrete hands-on ideas relating to all aspects of healthcare management, from strategic planning, operations, financial and human resource development, to dealing with providers and patients, and health information systems.

He brings into this book his thoughts and experiences from fighting in the "trenches" (wards and clinics) to executive boardrooms of healthcare institutions, towards delivering efficient, financially sound and sustainable quality of care, at various levels and settings. Like his earlier monograph with the late co-author Art Ouellette (2014), "An Investor's Guide to Developing a Private Hospital: Ten Considerations before Committing", this current volume contains pearls of wisdom, born out of his many years of health care administrative experience in the private sector and privatised public hospitals in Singapore and elsewhere all over the world."

Prof Phua Kai Hong
Visiting Professor
Graduate School of Public Policy
Nazarbayev University

Adjunct Faculty
Lee Kuan Yew School of Public Policy,
National University of Singapore, and Singapore Management University

Former Associate Professor and Head, Health Care Division,
Faculty of Medicine,
National University of Singapore

PREFACE

This book is based on a series of observations and anecdotes gained from my experience, exposure, research, and understandings gathered from working in healthcare systems of at least five different countries and compressed into "Reflections, Insights, and Lessons" statements for the purpose of being able to easily remember, but more importantly, share with you. Over the years, we have had the opportunity and privilege to *manage and be a Mentor* to a number of individuals who were recruited with related backgrounds in finance, operations, and other areas, and needed to be oriented and trained in application of their background within healthcare industry. Many of my "mentees" have risen, and assumed more senior roles, i.e. becoming CEOs/MDs, CFOs, and COOs who are now in the position to lead their respective organizations, and hopefully become Mentors as well, preparing future generations of healthcare professionals. For that reason we wish to assist and stimulate that process by sharing meaningful observations, with interested individuals.

Explanations follow each "Reflection, Insight, and Lesson" statement to provide context, background, or insight of the statements, and in certain instances, solutions considered and/

or adopted, to make them more meaningful. The Reflective observations shared here are applicable across the healthcare industry spectrum, both in the Private and Public sectors. Certain observations appear obvious, and may have already been addressed by a particular healthcare facility; however, most facilities, depending on geographic location are at different stages of development and maturity, ranging from pending/considering implementation, to various stages of completion. Further, given the number of Reflections, Insights and Lessons highlighted in this book, there will be information overlap in various instances, which is useful as it reinforces other statements, and provides consistency and continuity in what is being shared but balanced so as to avoid being boring.

Each Reflection, Insight, and Lesson shared in this book should become the basis for expanded thinking, generating additional ideas that can be applied as enhancements or modifications, specific to your organization, making the Reflection, Insight, and Lesson even more meaningful and relevant, while perhaps triggering a recall of similar memories and experiences you may have previously encountered.

Certain Reflections, Insights, and Lessons have relevance in other industries experiencing similar situations. I am confident many may have already been identified by other authors, motivational and management speakers; however, this compendium of selected observations for consideration relate specifically to the healthcare industry and may be more relatable to you, but all offer learning and "transfer of knowledge" opportunities to improve both your management skills and operational insight!

Initially, this book was targeted toward middle and more senior level healthcare management positions; individuals who have experience and can relate to various lessons and can reflect on them, as this lends credibility to other statements in the book which they have yet to experience; however, two additional targets have emerged.

My secondary target are "students" and others just entering the healthcare industry to give them a "flavor" of the types of situations that may occur, and complement any formal educational training they have received with realistic and practical insights.

The last, but not least target is the general public; those who are curious and have questions and/or want to learn more about what *drives* healthcare decisions, operations and practices within the industry. Even healthcare individuals and professionals may want more insight about various topics, to gain a better understanding and broaden their perspectives about operational responsibilities, as well as members of the journalistic and legal professions, and especially those who are contemplating undertaking healthcare projects.

The observations that form the basis of my Reflections. Insights, and Lessons have been "collected" during my years in healthcare having had the privilege to be appointed to lead roles of CEO, COO, CFO, at various healthcare facilities, and equally as many supporting roles. Many observations being shared were common in all the positions; others, were more focused to a specific role, but surprisingly, most are similar regardless of the countries worked in, i.e., US, Saudi Arabia, Philippines, Malaysia, China, Singapore, and India. We must also share there were times when we personally faltered and learned "hard lessons" but managed to recover and was made stronger. Therefore I am able to reflect upon and share many of the learning experiences with that legacy perspective so others can avoid making the same or similar mistakes. While I have been in the healthcare industry for many years, there are many more learned individuals, and those with more experience and insight from whom I can continue to learn, and respect.

Before we close off the Preface, I want to highlight three themes present in the book. The subtitle "*ProActive/ReActive*" connotes many of the Reflections, Insights, and Lessons are a result of proactive learning i.e., studying historical activities and reports, reading about different countries healthcare delivery systems, attending Conferences and Seminars on selected topics, networking with peers and being exposed to new concepts, able to discuss "best practices" and use of them to improve our performance. On the other side, many observations have their genesis in *Reactive* conditions, as result of internal or external questions, observed behavior, editorials, legal actions or situations that have challenged us and caused us to "think" of different solutions (sometimes out of the box) on ways to improve.

Another theme, I wish to focus upon is that of K*nowledge*. To be a successful Senior Administrator, one must take time to "learn the business" from the ground up. This does not mean one must have spent their entire career in healthcare, but it does mean the Administrator must take time to visit Departments in their organization and observe "front line" activities, to learn and develop an understanding and appreciation of what is happening which will allow Administrators to relate with and support their staff when difficult issues or questions arise. Interestingly enough in the process, through insightful questions Administrators can even identify archaic practices still in effect offering no "value add" that can be eliminated. If one is a Department Manager, learn everything you can about your business, treat it as if you were an independent "Owner-Operator" and your livelihood depended on it. As you move up the hierarchy, you should adopt the same principle but take on new, wider perspectives.

The final theme I want to mention is that of *Finance and Accounting*. At the most senior levels, everyone needs to have attended, at least, a basic Executive Level orientation course in accounting and finance so as to develop an understanding of key terms. Learn how to "read" a Profit and Loss Statement, Balance Sheet, and able to focus on the critical line items, ratios and metrics. Many financial and accounting terms will be used in the Board of Directors/Trustees Meetings, Budget preparation and reviews, and when sharing new concepts and ideas for implementation consideration, so as a Senior Administrator, avoid embarrassment regarding basic terminology and meanings. Your Chief Financial Officer, or equivalent, can take the lead when delving into details and financial reporting compliance; however understanding the basics both in the private and public sector is essential.

Whether you are a seasoned healthcare professional or just starting out on your middle to senior level healthcare administrative career, these observation based learning points about strategy, management, finance, and operations in the healthcare industry will be meaningful. The explanations offered provide "insights" which you can nurture, develop, and implement, but most of all, ENJOY!

Any comments, further elaborations, or sharing of different experiences are always welcome. Healthcare is a dynamic industry and requires continuous learning and upgrading by its professionals, at all levels. If we can assemble enough meaningful additional reflective observations and lessons, we can consider publishing a follow-up book in the future.

Steven J Sobak
September 2019

Contact: Sobak.Investor@gmail.com

Also by:

Arthur R Ouelette and Steven J Sobak, "An Investor's Guide to Developing a Private Hospital, Ten Considerations before Committing", (2014)

Dedication

To
Prof Cheng Heng Kock who encouraged me to collect, and share my experiences from over the years...........

And To
Theodore Gaston my first Mentor and Supporter in Healthcare

ACKNOWLEDGEMENTS

I would like to recognize the following individuals who took time from their respective busy schedules to read my draft versions and offer helpful and constructive comments, and support to improve understanding and interpretation. I have tried to incorporate all that I could.

(Mr) Boon Yeow Chew
(Dr) Jennifer Lee
(Dr) Yoong Siew Lee
(Dr) Eillyne Seow

And a Special Thanks to (Dr) Goh Hsin Kai for his clever Cover design and Illustrations

CONTENTS

PREFACE vii

We have divided the Reflective, Insight, and Lesson observations into four general categories; however, the content and placement within each category is subjective and I take responsibility for the selection. Even within categories, topics are "mixed" to keep the reading easy and hopefully interesting.

I   PATIENT RELATED OBSERVATIONS 1

II HEALTHCARE FACILITY RELATED
     OBSERVATIONS 35

III OPERATIONAL RELATED OBSERVATIONS 167

IV COMMON SENSE RELATED OBSERVATIONS ... 275

CLOSING 291

SELECTED TERMS AND DEFINITIONS
USED IN THE BOOK 293

SUBJECT INDEX 313

Characters of book

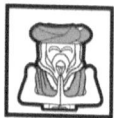
The Guru
*He is the "perfect one".........
a retired healthcare leader who has since achieved enlightenment*

The CEO aka boss
*He is the overall in charge of the system..........
always in shock, always stressed*

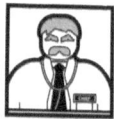
The Chief of doctors
*He is in charge of the doctors.........
cool headed but tired, retiring soon*

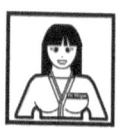
The young consultant, Dr HOPE
*She is a young specialist..........
dedicated, up and coming leader*

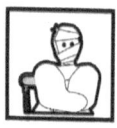
The Patient X
*He is a patient...........
saved by the hospital despite severe injuries*

PATIENT RELATED OBSERVATIONS

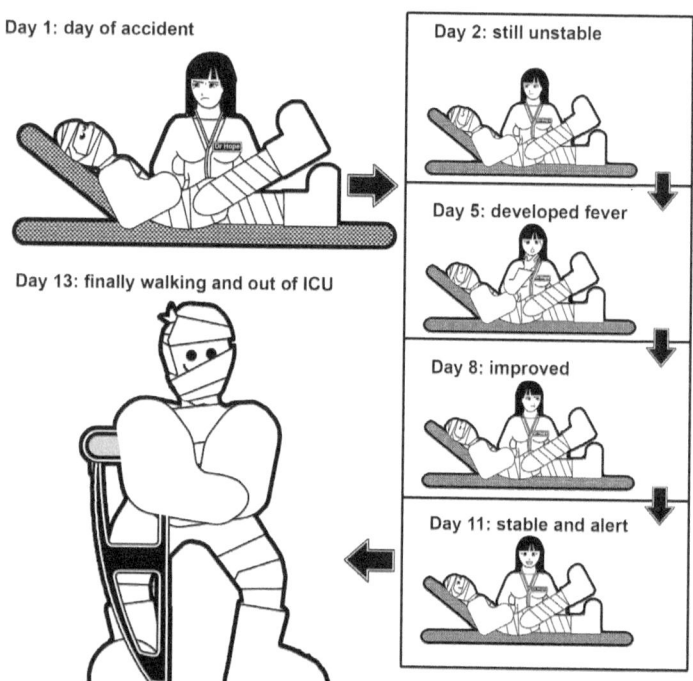

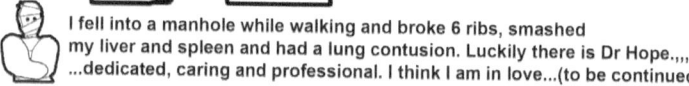
I fell into a manhole while walking and broke 6 ribs, smashed my liver and spleen and had a lung contusion. Luckily there is Dr Hope.,,, ...dedicated, caring and professional. I think I am in love...(to be continued)

1   Front line **professionals**, doctors, specialists, nurses, therapists and any other individuals interacting with the patients, **should demonstrate good hygiene practice, show interest, engage them,** making eye contact, talking to them (not at them), and asking "open ended" questions to obtain feedback from the patients on professionals understanding of their conditions, understanding of instructions given, and an understanding of what they want.

Unfortunately many patients meet with the Doctor, Specialist, Nurse or other service professionals, and after the meeting feel overwhelmed, or may fail to understand what transpired and what they need to do. This is particularly true for elderly, and patients who cannot communicate or interact with staff when medical services are being provided. So, use of body language, communication, visual supports (pictures, drawings, and pamphlets) should be the standard techniques used to engage the patients, caregivers, and family.

Doctors, Specialists and any staff who will be assisting, or touching any patient should make washing their hands before engaging the patient visible to the patient. Further, staff should look at the patient during the consultation or treatment, and avoid exclusively looking at the computer screen or writing without achieving eye contact with the patient. It is important to project interest in the patient's condition and making efforts in communication. Before closing off any Outpatient Clinical Attendance or Service Appointment, ask the patient, caregiver, family member to repeat the key tasks they need to perform, or symptoms that require immediate medical attention, to ensure they understand what was communicated. The best way is by using a series of "open ended" questions. If the patient cannot answer or has difficulty, then there is a problem that must be resolved before the patient leaves; otherwise they will be unable to convey what transpired or remember what they need to do after leaving the consultation room. Special instructions may need to be written down, or they be given a prepared instruction sheet to assist them in what to do. Ensure each patient facing staff is educated, "never allow a patient to leave their care without the patient/caregiver knowing what needs to be done, from taking medicine, to returning for follow-up service".

Similarly for inpatients, in addition to the above Observation points, all professionals (Specialists, Nurses, Therapists, etc.) should visit the patients, engaging the patients by asking certain "open ended" questions, specifically "How do you feel today", "How can I help you, to make you feel better", "What do you want or need", and listen to the responses, respond accordingly. Finally, take time to explain what activities and treatment plans are scheduled, and any changes that may occur for the day to keep them updated to manage their anxiety.

2. **Dress and Act like the professionals** we are supposed to be; then, we will be respected for who we are.

Doctors, nurses, therapists, administrators are all professionals in their respective areas of expertise. As such, the patients and their families have perceptions and expectations on how the professionals should be dressed, as well as generally accepted professional attire of the industry. Correct dressing promotes a professional image of the individual, and reflects on the standards of services being performed. Nurses often have healthcare facility specific standardized uniforms that they normally wear, and designed to be able to delineate their "rank", so this group is the easiest to identify in the organization, but even their uniforms need to be neat and tidy, especially when reporting to work. Understandably, during the course of the day they may get stained, but you can still tell they are part of the nursing team.

The attire of doctors over the years has been evolving. From a time where once the "white lab coat" was their trademark with a stethoscope around their neck, and having a bit of an antiseptic, clean smell from the frequent handwashing with germicidal soap to their current "wardrobe". Unfortunately, many "New generation" doctors wear conventional street clothes, and the only visible item to distinguish them as a doctor is their stethoscope, and normally a badge, making it difficult to differentiate them from patients, general staff, family or visitors. To further raise concerns and confusion, is that many of the newly minted doctors often look very young, so it is difficult for older patients, and their family/caregivers be comfortable in sharing and discussing certain personal, sensitive information and grasp that the youthful looking individuals are both trained and capable in managing their condition (perception management). Some doctors even come to work wearing clothes as if they came directly from a party or some other activity, which makes the situation more complicated. While medical staff dress code requirements may be changing, there should still be clear standards drawn up by the Medical Board, that all must comply to project a proper image of themselves and the important roles they perform, to promote confidence with the patients, caregivers, families, and organization to gain and be given the respect they deserve.

Clinical support staff (Lab Techs, Imaging, Pharmacists, Dieticians, Therapists, etc.,) tend to be the most identifiable as they all normally wear a Lab coat with their identification, so they meet most patients, and caregivers expectations as professionals.

Finally the administrative group must always be dressed conservatively, particularly those interacting and in direct contact with patients or their families to present a professional, and responsible appearance.

3   In the service related industry, a **SMILE**, is **Free** to **Give** and generates **INTEREST AND APPRECIATION** but "costs" much if saved, resulting in **DEPRESSION AND RECESSION**, primarily your own.

This observation is often given by patients while making complaints, particularly when they perceive they are being given less than the required level of attention they believe is deserved. How many times have we heard, "so and so always showing a black face"; "so and so does not acknowledge or recognize me, and I have been standing in front of them for so long"; "so and so begrudgingly gave me service and did not appear happy about it"; or many of variants of the same theme.

Basically we need to teach all the front line staff, or any staff having face to face contact with patients to display a more cheerful, but a situation appropriate, countenance. This includes all level of staff, from the clinical side (e.g., doctors, nurses, assistants, therapists, aides, pharmacists, imaging, etc.) as well as, all the support staff (e.g., patient transport, kitchen and meal attendants, drivers, housekeeping/environment, laundry, building maintenance etc.), all the way through to the Administrative staff (e.g., Admissions, Business Office, Registration and Front Desk, to Cashier, Human Resources, Finance, etc.).

We must never forget helping and treating patients are the reasons the healthcare facility is in operation, and we have a duty to provide the best care possible given the resources available. Patients must always "feel" they are appreciated, and given recognition regardless of the conditions that brought them to seek healthcare services. As such, we should make every effort to offer a simple but sincere smile, with a "how may I help you" attitude to start building a relationship, and communicating. Failure to make a simple connection will often result in negative feedback being given, and usually containing a litany of many other items causing dissatisfaction which will result in a substantial amount of time and effort from many parties to placate and salvage a relationship. In the meantime staff involved/tasked with investigating and preparing responses become frustrated and they become depressed – always seeing the negative side of people.

4   Always give a **Non-Attackable lead in explanation to any change**, it will reduce negative comments and facilitate the change.

Change is always difficult, and it is made more difficult if one fails to be tactful and considerate when attempting to provide an explanation. Being aware that the initial reaction of the individual(s) involved will most likely be defensive, it is important to provide proper explanations that are both logical and to which one can relate.

Often time, the opening lines of the conversation must be structured to allow for listening for any feedback before offering any explanations or background conditions leading up to the necessity for change. For example,

The organization tries to manage costs at "point of sale" locations. A decision is taken requiring items to be paid or settled at the checkout counter, rather than the organization billing for the services. Billing adds additional "backroom" costs to collect the money, as well as contributes to "bad debt" which then results in higher costs for the service or product. As the organization, wishes to manage costs for the benefit of the patients or customers, it is easier to convey the reason or rationale for the change and then seek to obtain their understanding, but it may take a longer time for people to appreciate the underlying principles and develop an acceptance. However, this type of change should be followed after highlighting different methods of payments the facility has made available, such as: cash, "tap" debit cards, credit cards, new cashless bank payment features, applications (apps) using smart phones and other devices so individuals can appreciate the efforts.

Once this is done, attempt to obtain "understanding" from the individuals by asking questions structured to develop a series of "yes" responses. "I am sure you do want the charges to be the lowest they can be?", "You do understand that it costs more to bill and send out statements, i.e. accounting, printing, postage, manpower, bad debt?".

Another example. I once had an elderly (80++) gentleman come storming into my office to complain about the high cost of the pacemaker recently implanted, stating the hospital was overcharging and trying to take advantage of the patient, government, or insurance, whoever was paying. After listening to him, I shared the hospital obtained specifications and features for pacemakers from the cardiologist specialists, and then called for quotes from reputable manufacturers offering a range of different models that met the clinician's needs. Qualified pacemaker brands and models were evaluated and made available to the Specialists for use in their procedures and ensure the best medical outcomes. After I listened to him and gave an explanation, I then asked him if he preferred a higher quality pace maker, versus a much lower priced one without features the Specialists wanted, or a pacemaker with marginal, poor, or unreliable outcome record for his implant. If the lower quality pacemaker failed to perform, then I told him "we would not be having this conversation". He finally left with the comments he was only concerned about the high costs, and wanted to ensure patients were fairly charged which we appreciated.

The same principles can be applied to making changes to policies and procedures within the organization, as they should always be to provide clarity, consistency, and standardization in performing tasks and managing most situations. Front line staff must be kept informed and provided with necessary background information and armed with a series of Questions and Answers (Q & As) developed in advance to facilitate responses.

The same approach can be used for both "face to face" conversations, as well as, written responses to any query, it just needs to be structured to lead and create understanding.

There may still be individuals who still have objections. If so, ask the individual(s) to provide alternative, practical solution(s) that satisfy their objectives leading to the changes but must be fair and equitable to all parties, and not just their special interests.

You may be surprised, and obtain some great ideas!!

5   Avoid **the use of negative words** (no, not, regret to say, cannot) as much as possible whenever responding to patient/customer feedback, and **PARTICULARLY** in the opening lines.

Be careful when responding to critical feedback by taking a defensive position too early. Often time we need to listen to the feedback, from individuals whether verbal or written. This has two effects, it allows for the individual providing the feedback to express their concerns from their perspective, and also allows us to obtain a better understanding of what the "real" underlying issue(s) may be. It is interesting that in many instances, there is an action or trigger point that caused the individual to take time to write in, and dismissing their feedback too early is both insulting and annoying to them, thereby creating an "air of superiority" on behalf of the respondents that usually results in escalation of the issue to a higher level. After listening to the feedback, and perhaps analysing what "message" is being conveyed, then it is the time to relate the information to the broader perspective. So in the conversation, whether a face to face discussion, or written text, it is important to share at least part of the rationale used for coming to a conclusion before making statements that are clearly negative in nature from their perspective.

If you are trying to educate or enlighten someone, use of negative terms too early causes the reader to mentally "turn off" with the impression that you are closed to listening; whereas, if after you have listened, then you can offer explanations to justify your position, or even acknowledge that the writer may have several good points that can and should be further explored and given proper consideration. Always try to share rationale for taking certain positions if they are contrary to what the feedback provider is trying to convey, While it may be impossible to change the individuals perspective, you have at least made an attempt to educate and have the individual also listen.

Only after taking the educational approach should you use any negatives terms to bring closure to the discussion, but always remember there may be legitimate points for consideration, and give the feedback provider acknowledgement of their "contribution" and that you will take the feedback seriously as policies and actions are being reviewed. There have been instances where the feedback proved to be valid and we did in fact make changes in the manner in which certain processes were performed, and we rewarded the individual with a "token" of appreciation.

6   Be Careful - Hospitals are one of the few places where it may be inappropriate to tell your customers/patients **"Hope to Serve/See you again – Soon!"** or **"Return Soon!"**

With Customer Service, Customer Relations, and Clinical Quality Standards in place the expectation is that the patient will achieve the objectives of an admission, and be discharged, with a positive experience. In most companies a satisfied "patient/customer/client" (however referred) will usually share their experience, which in turn generates referrals. However, unlike other industries, the healthcare industry tries to minimize repeat business for the same condition, except perhaps for obstetrics, and aesthetic services, so outwardly extending a wish to "see you soon, or return soon" may sometimes offend certain cultural sensitivities, as no one wants to be sick! This is true around the world. In fact, if returning too frequently some question the efficacy of the treatment being provided, apart for management of ongoing oncology (chemo-therapy), radiology (radio-therapy) treatments, and staged orthopedic operations/procedures.

So, while all healthcare providers (clinical, nursing, allied health, and other support services), want to be remembered for good service, it must be managed in a tactful manner, and the best measure of your staff's success is when patient's or their families make an effort to send a short letter, card, note and/or be given verbal and written feedback forms in appreciation of the care provided. Staff can also use this opportunity to give thanks to the feedback providers and share "you are there" should any situation arise in the future where your services are required. Use a soft, indirect approach!

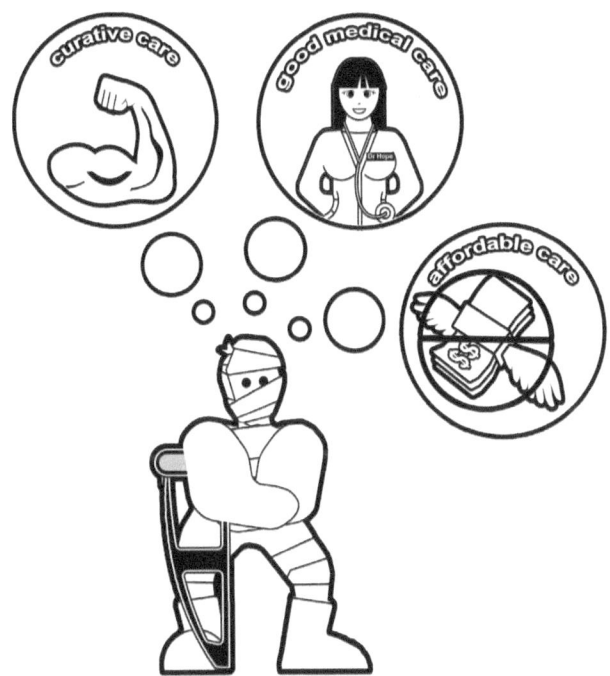

 Not all patients have a Dr Hope to help them, but all of them need hope!

7 A Hospital's primary service is the provision of **HOPE**.

7.1 **HOPE** to receive the best medical service possible.

7.2 **HOPE** to come out better and happier than when you went in.

7.3 **HOPE** that you do not have a "heart attack" when you receive the bill!

When a patient comes to hospital, it is a given that the individual will be treated with the best medical care available (this can vary immensely based on the hospital, specialties serviced, location, equipment, country, etc.) based on the presenting condition of the patient. Medical services could range from "heroic" surgical, life-saving procedures as a result of a trauma to aggressively treating a medical condition to save patients with serious illnesses, disease, infection with medication and drugs, therapy, or other acceptable treatments. Finally, it is important to provide compassion, and sensitive treatment during times of depression, and especially being sensitive to the patient's dignity during their final hours. What is always in the patient's and family mind is the Hope that the patient will achieve the best outcome possible. Survival with no "quality of life" is not a good outcome.

Based on statistics from various countries, most admitted patients are discharged, in a better condition than they entered; however, their "road to full recovery" is still a function of the long term care, attention and support given to the patient after discharge, and most importantly, the patient's personal commitment, and confidence to do what is necessary, and complete their course of treatment. If done, in most instances the patient will actually be in better condition and "spirits" than when they were admitted. One must recognize given the admitting condition, better is a relative comparison, and does not necessarily connote they will be equal to or better than they were before the event that triggered their admission, but they have achieved a state where they are able to live the best they can. Several examples come to mind. After a severe accident, a patient is brought to hospital after sustaining severe trauma, such as loss of a limb. The hospital will manage the treatment of the limb loss, but the patient will need to undergo "rehabilitation" either within the same or another hospital, as an outpatient, and at home with assistance from the family or caregiver. Another instances would include patients who suffered a heart attack, stroke, debilitating neurological condition (ALS, etc.), or infection. Once the condition is stabilized, surgery performed if necessary, medication given, the patient starts the recovery process. Suffering from these types of conditions, will most likely require short to long term medication and lifestyle changes to achieve recovery and live with dignity.

In both these instances, efforts are to demonstrate the patient received the best care/treatment possible with available resources, and discharged in a stable or better condition than what they were in at the point of admission.

Finally, it is also important to choose the level of care a patient or family can afford to avoid a shock or surprise (figuratively- heart attack) when they receive the bill. Another example, normally when a woman comes to deliver, this is a "happy" event and the husband and/or family want her to enjoy the experience, so may admit her to a Class of Service or accommodations at a higher standard than what they can normally afford as the expected stay is only for one to four days. If the delivery goes as planned, with no complications, indeed the event would be memorable in a positive way. However, if the neonate experiences some complication e.g. prematurity, congenital heart condition, or even jaundice, it may require the neonate to be admitted at one of the Neonatal Intensive Care Units (NICUs), following the class and fee standard the mother chose. Typically the cost of staying in any NICU is several multiples of a normal stay, so depending on how long the neonate's admission lasts and treatments required, it will determine the size of the bill, based on the mother's Class of Admission. This bill can become relatively substantial, and give the poor parents quite a shock and turn a "happy" event into a time of stress.

It has been proven with proper information, parents are able to better plan the admissions and services at prices they could afford, so the principle of Financial Counseling, was introduced, sharing the various levels of projected Bill sizes based on the Class of Service/Standards selected. After implementation, expectation mismatching went very low. Subsequently, no more "heart attacks" when the family received the bill. Hospital bills could still be large, but manageable with proper planning and selection of services.

8. For any formal response to a contentious letter or issue addressed to CEO (or equivalent), **it is wise to have the initial response be signed off by a direct report individual familiar with the issue after discussion with CEO** on the possible outcomes and strategy. This allows for the CEO to function as the "appeal individual" who has the authority to either support, or modify, the initial response outcome should conditions merit, lest the issue be raised up to a higher level (HQ or Board) for resolution. Normally, HQ or the Board will refer the issue back to CEO to prepare the reply, and/or meet with the aggrieved party(ies) since they will not have the necessary information.

Whenever a letter relating to a complaint or issue was addressed **directly** to the CEO/MD by name, we employed a specific internal strategy when responding keeping in mind an important principle - one must always leave an avenue for appeal. Understanding if CEO/MD signs off on the initial response, then the recourse for the individual raising the complaint/issue is normally to escalate their appeal to another level, such as a Board Member, Headquarters, or the Health Ministry/Department. So, in most instances, effort is made to contain the responses within the Senior Operational (Chief, or Director) levels of the organization rather than getting Board Members or others involved, as in most cases they are not familiar with the detailed operations, and will usually delegate the response down to the CEO/MD to manage and reply.

To minimize this from occurring, the COO and/or Service Quality staff would "do the homework" by investigating the feedback and expectation, then prepare a draft response. COO would then meet and update CEO/MD about the facts, review the proposed response, as well as consider possible outcomes to the reply (i.e., accept, disagree, appeal, etc.) and then issue the letter on behalf of CEO/MD signed by COO. In many instances, complaints are without merit and more a "matter of perception", as the standard is that all actions taken or services provided by the organization should be documented as part of the Medical Record. The response to the writer would be crafted offering the information to address the issues raised; however, at times the writer would refuse to accept the reply and continue to disagree or again appeal to the CEO/MD. Should this occur, we would then reconsider the situation and assess our position, as well as, the potential time cost, effort, and other factors that could arise, e.g. negative media, PR. As long as there were no medical or ethical issues involved, after discussion, a decision could be taken citing CEO/MD has reconsidered the appeal, by reversing part or all of the earlier items/issues in contention, and becomes "good guy". In most cases where this occurred, this approach closed the particular episode without the issues being escalated.

It is critical to always have a "Plan B" to manage an appeal. In most cases, feedback complaints usually are received by the formal or informal channels, such as Service Quality, Patient Affairs, Department Heads, feedback forms, survey, or other written or verbal feedback channels available. Responses and information gathering is normally coordinated by the Service Quality Section (or equivalent) along with mandatory input from the Department Head where the alleged shortcoming(s) occurred. This approach is so the Department Head is aware of issues arising in areas under their supervision, can explore and rectify as required. This approach also allows an avenue for appeal to any of the Senior Chief level positions as necessary.

9. Interesting how it is only the **FINAL REMINDER** that ever reaches the patient, when there has been no change in any particulars.

After a patient is discharged from hospital, ambulatory outpatient care, emergency services, or clinics, and there are outstanding balances that need to be settled, the organization sends out the bill with the outstanding amount. If not settled within 30 days, a first notice is sent out, and subsequently a second reminder is sent out after 60 days. Normally after reaching 90 days a "final" reminder is sent out with an indication that the bill will be transferred to a "bill collection" service" for continued follow-up and settlement. Ironically, many times patient's or relatives will respond to the third and final reminder, either sending in payment or stopping at the Business Office Cashier claiming they never received the earlier bills or notices, when all the billing particulars and address are the same. When billings are submitted to the Collection Agency, several actions can take place. More aggressive, but not "harassing" follow-up is performed, and the organization has the option and right to notify the Credit Agency of the delayed or delinquent payment which could impact on their future credit rating. We have assessed this situation that individuals or families respond to the Third reminder for both the perceived action of the Collection Agency and equating it to Loan Shark tactics, potential damage to their credit rating, and acceptance that the organization is not "forgetting" about the outstanding amount, so best to settle the outstanding balance.

10. Note that the perceived value of services rendered, and the **number of shortcomings encountered** are in direct proportion to the "cash out of pocket" amount remaining on a patient's bill; however, their remedy is often found in the amount of waiver offered.

Related to delayed or delinquent payments, individuals will lodge complaints on services they perceived failed to meet their expectations. Often, when someone is ill or involved in an accident, the individual or immediate family will express the hospital staff should do all that is necessary to help the patient and they will undertake the expenses. However, there are times when the reason given for delayed or non-payment is "justified" by a litany of complaints of actual/perceived shortfalls in service expectations and not addressed while receiving treatment. In most instances they relate to interpersonal skill, rather than actual medical treatment. The individuals will claim the doctor or nurses had "black faces", did not smile, did not appear to be interested in the patient or otherwise preoccupied, or a specific supply, consumable, or medication was not given to them on a certain day and time, food and physical ambiance were not up to their expectations. The litany length of complaints is usually in direct proportion and size of the outstanding balance to be settled. What they are looking for is a partial concession, or discount from the charges, to complete waiver of the outstanding balance for the actual/perceived shortcomings. Since this is being presented well after the discharge, it is difficult to ascertain the validity of all the details as they are listed, so a more general approach is usually taken. After reading or listening to the feedback, an agreement can usually be reached to reduce or waive certain items as a compromise, if they agree to settle the remaining portion of the outstanding bill immediately. This approach normally works, but the amount or percentage has to be a negotiated amount and is usually a function of the size of the bill. As this bill has been outstanding for a considerable amount of time, and depending on the amount involved, it requires a decision of how much additional time and effort is to be expended to reach a settlement, file a claim, or other legal action to close the account. The adjustments were never for the medical services or treatments rendered. If the patient complained about the medical treatment, that automatically elevated the discussion to another level involving medical staff as their allegations become potential medical-legal issues. We never compromise on medical treatment. All other complaints are looked at holistically, and certain line items may be adjusted out of the bill or a general discount of "x" percent may be negotiated; but in all my years, these discounts, to my recollections, never exceeded 15% of the outstanding bill for non-clinical items, and most were in the range of 5-8%. The question arises from a business perspective of how much does the institution want to spend and delay settlement for a relatively small concession.

An interesting exercise is to calculate amounts for potential waiver consideration by performing a "costing" of all the time spent in crafting response letters, vetting, rewriting, and review. Depending on the issues, collect the time of staff spent to investigate, review Medical Records, validate, calibrate, as well as, time contributions of Doctors, Specialists or Senior Administrative staff consulted or involved in review of ten to twenty responses for each of three response tiers of letters, specifically: simple, moderate complexity, and complex. This will give a range of cost to reply for each tier, and can be used as a gauge/proxy of an amount that could be waived for certain legitimate feedback. The amounts defined can be delegated to staff at different levels, empowering them to resolve certain issue(s). For example, if an individual patient claims that a particular supply, medication, or service was not performed, and the cost of the item(s) involved are relatively low, and a quick review of the records fail to capture it being documented, we would give the patient "benefit of doubt" and waive the amount, rather than engage in a "war of words", and creating negative goodwill out of the situation. Applying the tier structure to the case, it could also be used to validate the reasonableness of a discount/waiver amount under consideration.

You would be surprised to learn how much time and cost is involved in preparing a response! However, this cost component is only one aspect to be included in the investigating and responding to feedback complaints involving requests for adjustments.. Use this approach as a "tool".

11   It is amazing that after almost 30 years, there are still **people who claim "they have not heard of"** MediSave, MediShield, or MediFund (In Singapore Context).

Starting back in 1986, and through 2000 Singapore introduced several healthcare "safety nets" to help Singaporeans manage their healthcare costs. The first one was *MediSave*, and was financed by a contribution of 6% from the individuals Central Provident Fund (CPF) account, set aside for the individual/immediate family's use to settle inpatient hospitalization bills, and certain selected outpatient managed conditions or procedures. While this approach to plan for one's healthcare needs is applicable in the Singapore environment, there may be similar structures available in other countries or organizations. Subsequently *MediShield* was introduced to serve as a high level insurance coverage with the premiums paid from the individuals CPF account contributions to help settle very expensive procedures within the Public and Private sector Hospitals. There are "caps" on the amounts that can be used, but the coverage substantially reduces the individual or family exposure to very expensive treatments or procedures, such as heart transplants, open heart surgery, lung related surgeries, brain surgery, chemo-therapies, stem cell transfusion, various joint replacement procedures, and rectification of congenital conditions to name a few. Since *MediSave* has been implemented, many individuals have obtained their necessary treatment, at a much reduced cost.

Finally *MediFund* was set up as a Government Funded "Trust Fund", in which the interest from the Fund's principle is used to assist needy, but eligible individuals in Government/Public hospitals without financial means to settle their healthcare bills. It serves as a "safety net" and citizens should appreciate and not feel shy to seek assistance in times of need. Culturally, many senior citizens often "feel shy, or embarrassed" to indicate they need help and end up waiting too long and their body subsequently suffers from multi-organ system failure, which is avoidable.

The "Medi-Series" of services were implemented to assist individuals. While it cannot provide 100% coverage from "cradle to grave" is offers many features to lessen the financial burden on the population when they need medical services. So after many years (since 1986) this message should be communicated to all citizens.

12. When trying to resolve financial issues, ensure you **identify the "drivers/causes" of the problems**, and not merely address the symptoms.

This is the administrative corollary to the medical practice of understanding the symptoms of a presenting problem and ultimately identifying the "root cause" and resolving the issue on a permanent basis. While the problem may present as an operational, or financial issue, it may actually have its actual "roots" in a medical practice, so all parties may need to work closely together.

A good example was shortly after the restructuring of Singapore General Hospital in Singapore, the CFO was inundated with many appeals directly from patients and via Member of Parliament (MP) Letters requesting to reduction of bills for families whose babies ended up having to stay in Neonatal Intensive Care Unit (ICU) after delivery for various complications, ranging from jaundice to other congenital conditions, some of which required substantial amount of time to rectify, e.g. prematurity, heart conditions, herniated conditions, etc. What was expected to be a "happy event" turned into a nightmare for some families who normally would not have selected a Private Class accommodations and treatment, but chose to do so for the happy event, which normally requires about a two to three day stay in hospital. When the baby was delivered with a condition requiring hospitalization, the baby was admitted, and charged the ICU rate based on the mother's selected Class of Accommodation and service, so the family started being billed at Private Class ICU rates which were substantially higher than Subsidized services available, (in the range of two to three times or higher based on the services required). As a result of the influx of requests for downgrade and waivers of the substantial bills, the "root cause" of the dilemma was evaluated to be an incorrect choice of service, which was outside the financial wherewithal of the family for an extended stay.

Once this was identified, the concept of bill size Financial Counseling was introduced to assist Obstetric patients. As Admission staff were not privy to the financial particulars of any family, the Finance and Business Office Staff, with guidance, were tasked to create a simple template to explain the different fee structures associated with the three/four different Classes available. The resultant template design disclosed implications and potential financial burdens to expect by choosing different Private versus Subsidized Care Classes, should either the newborn or mother need to be admitted should any complication(s) arise. Information was presented to the family as an Average Bill Size (ABS) for each Class of Service for both normal length of stay, and at the 80-90 percentile level so the parents could take an informed decision on which Class of Service they could comfortably manage (in a worst case situation) given their family's financial resources.

With introduction of this simple practice, the number of appeals for waiver or downgrade consideration essentially went to "zero". The only instances to occur after adopting this practice were the few individuals/families who still opted for the higher Private Class Accommodations after Financial Counselling, and there was a complication. Since they were properly counselled, alternative settlement options for these cases were offered to assist, but not waived.

Due to the success of the ABS Financial Counseling for Obstetric patients, Finance and Business Office expanded the scope of the Financial Counseling to other selected medical conditions and procedures with similar good outcomes in management of patient's expectations by selecting medical/surgical services within their financial means. Subsequently the concept was adopted by all the Government Restructured Hospitals, and finally extended and made mandatory for all Hospitals in Singapore both Government/Restructured and Private. Over the years the simple paper based templates were replaced with more sophisticated presentations relying on regularly updated Average Bill Size billing information for specific procedures (using DRGs). Finally, new software was developed for use at the Admission Offices, and over the years the process has been further refined into a Financial Counseling Application (App) accessible at home for patients to complete their mandatory Financial Counselling before admission. This reduced pressure on taking the decision at Admission time, and allows the family to discuss their choices.

While this story is long, it demonstrates how a recurring financial issue for patients and families was investigated, identifying the "driver, or root cause" of the problem and responding with a creative, workable, new solution which effectively eliminated the appeals and MP Letters, as well as benefiting all patients being admitted to hospital in the future.

13   Most patients or parents fail to appreciate the **value of a doctor's Clinical Assessment/Information** shared at a Consult, and measure the "quality of service" by how many tests are ordered, procedures performed, and/or number of prescriptions written.

In certain countries and cultures, when patients seek medical services, either with a General Practitioner (GP) or Specialist, there is an expectation the doctor will order a battery of tests, e.g. laboratory, images, etc. to ascertain the medical condition of the patient before they determine the procedures to be performed, treatments, and medication to be given for the presenting condition. Based on a good history taking of the patient's condition, many illnesses do not require an extensive battery of tests for the doctor to recognize the symptoms of a particular disease, and the doctors can provide the patient or family with an explanation.

Unfortunately, many families believe there is a correlation between the number of tests performed, images taken, prescriptions given and the diagnosis of the patient. If the doctor fails to meet their expectation, then they equate the service provided as incomplete.

So, in many instances when parents take their child(ren) to a doctor at a government owned and operated public General Practitioner (GP) Polyclinic facility, or even at a Specialists Clinic in a hospital, the doctors may recognize the presenting symptoms, and will provide an explanation, offer advice, then send the child home. However, the family may then seek out a private doctor, who will order a battery of tests for the patient, offer some medications to help relieve the symptoms, and the parents end up paying two to three or more times the amount than charged at the Government facility. During this time, if the child had a virus, it will normally resolve itself after five to seven days, but the parents will equate the recovery with the tests and symptomatic relief medications given and not the fact the disease has "run its course". Doctors spend many years learning, and treating patients so they can recognize most emerging medical conditions by the presenting symptoms supported by an accurate medical history without the need for so many tests to determine an underlying cause, so their advice should be appreciated.

In contrast, there are other countries where parents and patients find comfort in the doctor's assessment of the condition, with a good "layman term" explanation by the doctor/specialist, and assurance the patient will recover within a specific time period, with instruction to monitor the condition, and take further action only if the condition deteriorates. In the meantime, the patient can return home. Money for all the tests and investigations can be saved, and this helps to keep overall healthcare costs manageable.

14   In a healthcare setting (hospital, clinic etc.), always remember **"if it is not documented, it is not done"**.

For both the patient as well as the organization this simple statement can have substantial impact. There have been many instances when a patient, insurance company (as part of an audit), or whoever is legally responsible for settlement of the patient's account queries about charges for specific procedures performed, medications provided, or services billed. The hospital or healthcare facility typically needs to perform a review of the patient's medical record looking for supporting documentation entries that the service was properly ordered, as well as documentation it was provided. If there is proper documentation, it is easier to justify and explain the charge to the patient or justify the claim to the insurance company. However, if there is a lack of documentation for any service ordered and/or delivered, then it becomes difficult to justify the charge. Normally it results in giving the patient the "benefit of doubt" and making an adjustment to the bill or issuing a refund. If it was discovered during an insurance audit of bills they paid on behalf of their clients, they will calculate an amount based on net of "overbilled less under billed" amounts and claim reimbursement.

This lack of documentation in proper chronological sequence for an inpatient stay, or outpatient visit creates a situation whereby the organization may suffer a shortfall in money if the service was actually performed; however, if the charges are incorrect then this may lead to an internal investigation if it appears to be more than random events. In both instances, managers and staff providing services must be reminded to ensure any services provided are properly documented. NOTE: Accurate documentation is also critical in cases where legal action has been initiated, and pending investigation. The same principles apply, and could have substantial medical-legal implications.

One approach used to address the issue was to establish a "chart audit" function whereby a Chart Auditor (Accounting and/or Nursing background) compared selected detailed patient bills, meeting specific criteria, against the detailed patient's medical record looking for discrepancies, either over or under reporting, of services rendered, or lack of documentation for charges generated. A report was generated, sent to CFO for appropriate action. The documentation improved awareness of the situation and the percentage of errors reduced. With the improved collections, and saving of refunds, the cost of the FTE(s) was more than justified!

Remember, efforts must be made to ensure patients are never charged incorrectly as part of a proper service culture, and the healthcare organization should never suffer a loss of revenue for actual services rendered.

15   As professionals, we must convey to patients an **ER/A&E is operated on a 24 x7 basis** and evaluates patients on a **"triage basis"** to establish treatment priority **rather than a "first come, first serve" basis.** So, expect there may be "waiting time" incurred for less serious conditions.

Individuals seeking treatment in an Emergency Room or Accident & Emergency Department (ER/A&E) are treated after each patient is reviewed by a "triage" nurse or other qualified individual, doctor or paramedic. Basic vitals and information is taken from all the patients seeking treatment, to determine who has the most serious or "life threatening condition", head trauma, accident trauma, resuscitation condition, extensive burn, or major infectious condition, etc., will be given priority, over anyone with a simple cough and cold, minor injury, or allergic reaction, who will need to wait until the more serious medical cases are resolved. Depending on the day, time and activity level, waiting time could be only a matter of minutes or up to three or four hours. While waiting, a nurse will normally circulate to observe all patients, and determine if anyone's condition has deteriorated, which could justify moving them up on the priority scale.

Recognizing most patients or family's member who bring in a patient to the ER/A&E believe their situation is critical; whereas, the Triage staff are specially trained and experienced in assessing "presenting conditions" to establish treatment sequencing. To facilitate, hospital management can take various efforts and initiatives to manage patient/family expectations, such as,

15.1 Posting an "Average Waiting Time" at or near the entrance to inform individuals arriving at the ER/A&E.

15.2 Assigning/Calling back additional Specialist(s), and support doctors staff during days and peak hours over the week, based on patient activity profile or responding to external emergency situations.

15.3 Adding more treatment/examination rooms,

15.4 Performing certain procedures in preparation of being treated by the Specialist, e.g., any diagnostic Imaging or Lab test,

15.5 Introducing Observation beds in or near the ER/A&E to hold and observe conditions with intermittent symptoms.

15.6 Having an internal policy that after waiting "x" hours, will upgrade the individual to minimize further waiting.

15.7 Opening a general GP Clinic at or near the ER/A&E, staffed by GP(s) to facilitate in identifying the patient's condition, treat minor conditions, provide medication, and assist in obtaining a Specialist appointment if necessary. Depending on popularity and availability, the Clinic can also be expanded to provide a travel or employment vaccination service.

15.8 Liaising with local external GPs near the hospital on their hours of operations and provide information at the ER/A&E counter and should the patient or family decide to seek alternative service.

It is important to note, most doctors or nurses will avoid telling anyone to leave, lest something happen while in transit; however most individuals will "get the message" that their condition may not be so serious if given a longer waiting time.

So, the message is that Management needs to convey is, "use the services appropriately to everyone's benefit", as this will allow for treatment of critical cases in a timely manner, yet at the same time be creative in options to manage patient flow, and sensitive to waiting time. Also bear in mind that up to 25-40% of Hospital admissions can come through the ER/A&E, so it is an important portal, and requires serious attention! Given the 24x7 operational nature of an ER/A&E, it will always be expensive for a consultation and potential treatment, so help to contain costs.

16 Remember, **never immediately send out a reply to negative criticism, comment, or story**, as it is often written in a reactionary, emotional "state of mind". Allow at least 24-48 hours to lapse before sending out, after regaining both composure and an objective mindset. However, if one must respond on short notice, have the reply vetted by individual(s) not directly involved to ensure the reply content is accurate, tone is correct, and addresses the facts or issues raised. Otherwise, you will only make the situation more complicated.

There are instances where negative criticism is received, either directed to a specific individual, or a generalization. It is normal for feeling and sensitivities to be offended. Depending on the situation and individuals involved, one must exercise control of immediately responding when frustrated or hurt by any insensitive comments. Therefore it is important to allow for a "cooling down" period, and also try to understand the reasons for the critique, and if there is a real basis for the complaint. Remember, in any service industry, "perception is reality" with patients and general public, so take time to assess the situation, and then prepare a draft response, addressing the situation. It may even be appropriate to invite the writer to meet and provide further clarification in an attempt to discuss and resolve the situation amicably.

Should the decision be to write back without any contact, then it is important to be objective in the response and ensure it addresses the key points, or underlying concerns. But before that, take time to gather information (verbal and written) to document and gather facts from the hospital's perspective. This information can be used in crafting the response. Note in certain instances, it may be better to answer in a general context rather than a "point for point" response if there is a general pattern of overall dissatisfaction over relatively minor issues; however, you must use your best judgement and make that call, otherwise you could escalate the emotions of the writer.

Final word of advice is to have one or two staff, not directly involved, read both the negative feedback/criticism, and the proposed reply to determine if the issues were in fact addressed, and if the response is appropriate, and not inflammatory. Keep in mind, there will be instances where whatever communication is provided, the feedback writer will fail to accept the response and may escalate their concerns so be prepared.

HEALTHCARE FACILITY RELATED OBSERVATIONS

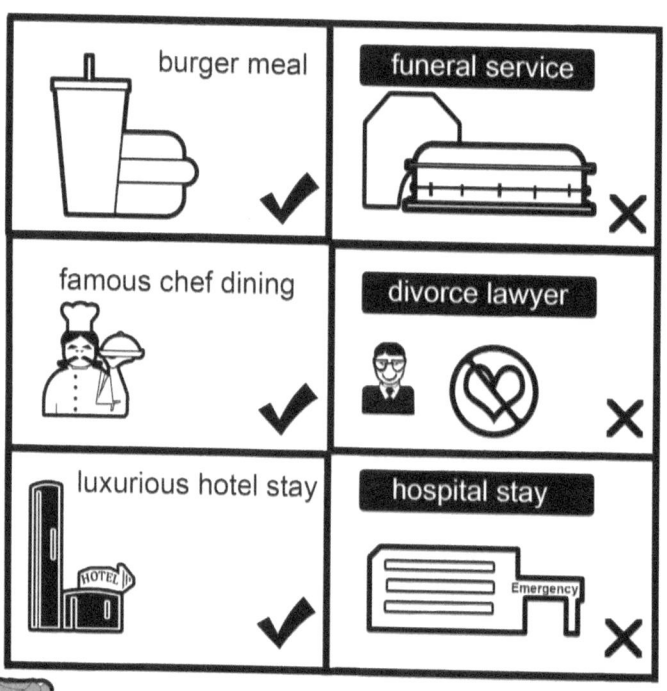

One for One marketing will simply not work in some industries

1   **Difficult to offer "frequent flyer" type recognition** to patients in healthcare. Consider, "have two surgeries, get the third for free", "remove one (part) for full price, the second for half price", "so many days and admissions at lower class accommodations (B2/C), get a free upgrade to private, (A/B1) Class". (Singapore, and other countries following a tiered inpatient structure)

As an organization, we are always looking to the "best practices" of other industries to determine which may be applicable and adaptable to the hospital and healthcare industry. The Frequent Flyer concept offering special services as discounted multi-procedure price packages, do not auger well with patients seeking healthcare services, as in most cases they are ill and not is a good mood. Wishing patients well at time of discharge is very good, but not the wish to see them back at hospital soon, this is taken as having very negative connotations.

While the medical services must be managed sensitively there is nothing preventing improved services to the patients and relatives to make their interactions more positive particularly for patients coming back for frequent treatments, such a hemodialysis, chemo and radiation therapies, rehabilitation (occupational, physical, speech, respiratory) etc. These groups of "frequent flyers" can be given special attention, such as fast track registration and payments/billings, special waiting areas, selected appointment times to make their visits more memorable. Offering room upgrades (in private or government hospitals) on a "space available" basis for patients requiring frequent admissions can be managed and considered. Whatever special privileges may be selected, they should be easy to administer, and avoid complicated processes with require substantial dedicated staff.

2   Observation. Why is it that whenever the Higher Level(s) of an organization decides to become leaner and more efficient, this translates into "pushing down/delegating" duties it used to perform, and the Middle Level gets larger, while **the Higher Level never seems to decrease on a permanent basis**, and the Lower (Operational) Levels incur more overhead cost, and activity answering to multiple "Heads or Levels"…?

This is an interesting anomaly. So many times over the years in different organizations there have been major reorganizations or restructuring both in the public and private sectors with the view to become more "lean and mean", reduce cost, and be more efficient by allowing for decisions to be made "closer" to where the action is occurring. The reorganizations normally result with an objective to "push down" many corporate level duties to mid-level operations, or directly to the facilities, which may result in the opening or closing of regional offices, with expectation that there will be reductions in the Corporate Headquarter/Ministry offices and related manpower, by consolidating functions. While it looks good on paper the reality of the situation is that this will work for a period of time. In the meantime responsibilities will be passed down to facilities, to be absorbed by existing staff until it reaches a point where all the requirements cannot be satisfied by the intermediate levels. So the Corporate or Regional Centers will start to add positions again to perform required tasks, and soon the positions initially reduced will return with different titles and focus.

This works well during "good times" but become more problematic during economic downturns, so there must be a clear objective with defined metrics to measure the before and after results to determine the success of the initiatives. Metrics can be both "hard", i.e. actual financial saving/redistribution of funds, reduction of staff, or "soft" i.e. improvement in service response, reduction in complaints, faster approval and evaluation of new programs, reduction of "bureaucratic "red tape". If this occurs then the initiative was meaningful.

However, the "downside" to the process is that Management in the Institutions or Facilities start to consolidate power and authority; however, if the Boards/Ministries perceive a loss of control or observe "silo" mentalities developing and positioning themselves for more power, they will intervene by taking back roles in the name of "better coordination". So, be mindful and ensure all aspects are considered for both the short and long term implications.

3   As part of Senior Management, if you want to know what is really happening in the Institution/Facility, **you need to walk around the place to observe.** Take time each week to observe the condition of the facilities, equipment, and staff. When you ask Heads of the Department, you will receive a partial answer. When you ask the ground staff, they will always say "all is fine" as they do not want to embarrass

their Supervisor. So to "give face" to all, observe for yourself!

We have all heard the saying "we need to walk the talk" to be credible, and this is really important in the healthcare setting. As senior management (CEO, COO, CFO, or their equivalents) we must take time to walk around our facilities on a regular basis, be visible, be aware, observe and know what is actually happening "on the ground". While we expect our direct reports and key management staff to ensure "everything is working properly", we also need to periodically satisfy ourselves that what is said is actually occurring. While I was serving at different facilities, I made it a habit in walking to different parts of the hospital, one or more Department areas on a weekly basis and was accompanied by the Head of Environmental/Housekeeping Services, Head of Facility Engineering, and Maintenance, and one or two junior staff to inspect each area selected for that week to learn and take notes on items requiring attention. Once in the specific inspections area, the Team would look closely into the condition of items under their responsibility, recorded deficiencies, or shortcoming, and were tasked with resolving problems over the next week. We even organized "SWAT" Teams. One or more teams of staff who performed focused tasks in Housekeeping areas, such as; "Hi-jetting" areas where there was a build-up of mold, dirt; special cleaning of "waste/bin collections" areas; stairs; floor polishing and buffing; toilet condition inspection and testing of faucets, drains, water pressure, mold build-up, and shower rail positioning; pest control; cleanliness in the kitchen and food preparation, serving and distributions systems; etc. Additional teams were organized by Facility Engineering, and Maintenance, covering all facility related conditions that needed attentions, such as; inspections of all drainage pipes in the wards and clinics; repairs of privacy curtain rods; doors and bumper rails; repair or replacement of tiles; repairs or replacement of patient beds and bedside tables; concrete flooring, and sidewalks; inspection of electrical and wiring issues; locate formal and informal storage areas used to collect defective, inoperative, or calibration overdue equipment on the wards and treatment areas, and had the items removed, etc. to minimize risk of the items being used on patients. These special activities all evolved as a result of performing "walk arounds" within the facilities when working as CFO and COO. This helped raise the standards and the cleanliness all around the facility and grounds. We always made an effort to keep "walk arounds" on a specific day and time so everyone was able to plan accordingly. With the key staff as part of the exercise, tasks and assignments were "easy" to assign, and faster than requests going through "channels". Staff were also tasked to continue the process even when CFO was unavailable due to a pressing meeting or unplanned situation.

Another excellent outcome of the process was that the Team had the opportunity to meet most of the staff throughout the organization, from the first line staff through Department Supervisors and Managers, and they all became comfortable with talking and sharing information and ideas with my "Walk Around" Team. We knew the condition of the facility, and were able to take proactive and pre-emptive actions to resolve issues, and give the front line staff support. As part of my "walk around", we even questioned Managers on their working standards and workload performance levels for the day/week/month to encourage and develop them by taking ownership of their areas.

So the task of walking around and learning the facility from the ground up is a critical function that either the COO or CFO should routinely perform, and include the CEO when time permits.

4   **Hospital beds**, in many locations, are like closets, the more you have, **the more to fill-up**!

This phenomenon occurs under two distinct environments, but for different reasons.

In developed countries, the bed utilization metric is "percentage of bed occupancy" which normally follows a "bell shaped" curve "life cycle", with lower occupancy numbers as a new facility opens up, approaches optimum bed occupancy range as it establishes a positive service reputation, and attracts a following of respected specialists who attract patients, and finally may decline over time due to new technologies, or change in patient profiles. Keep in mind the percentage of bed occupancy level is a function of at least three key variables, specifically, medical specialty, Length of Stay (LOS), and workload demand. For an extended period of time, bed occupancy will hover in the optimal 60-85+% range of the hospital's bed capacity. If a sustained high end occupancy pattern (86-90%++) occurs, it may justify expansion by conversion of support service areas to wards, adding a new floor/wing or even a new facility on the same grounds or nearby town/community to accommodate the increased workload. Management (Ministries/Boards) must be particularly sensitive to the medical specialties in demand, changes in technologies (new drugs, treatment protocols, procedures, robotics, AI, etc.), and shifts in treatment patterns (inpatient to day treatment, to outpatient, to home health care services) to sustain optimal utilization of the facility that will have an impact on inpatient bed demand, and reduce Lengths of Stays (LOS) for specific Specialties.

In under-developed or developing countries, where there is a shortfall of hospital beds and where general accessibility to basic medical care is limited or widely dispersed, there will be a greater need. If either government or private sector hospitals are built, they will attract patients to a point where they are filled, requiring additional beds which will fill-up, and perpetuate the cycle, assuming there is funding until a saturation point is achieved.

However, the limiting factor under both environments is availability of qualified staff, particularly doctors, specialists, and nursing personnel which can be a substantial operational hurdle. Additional Allied Health staff (laboratory, imaging, pharmacy, therapy services) will be needed to allow for expansion and complementing both acute/chronic inpatients as well as outpatient medical services provided.

Over time the demographic profile of the community or area being served by the hospital(s) will change, so the facilities will accordingly need to modify medical services offered to continue being meaningful. Failure to do so will result in consolidation or closing.

So, the more beds opened and available to accommodate the service area, the more beds will be filled-up with patients, both from the need, as well as availability basis; so carefully monitor and manage bed utilization and ALOS accordingly, with sufficient justification, and comprehensive current and forward planning. The more "closet" space one has the more to store, the more hospital beds available, more to fill-up.

A complementing step to manage the proliferation of beds, and their "filling up" is the educational aspect. The community must be educated to use the facilities wisely. Often time, the mindset is to seek services of specialists in the tertiary level care hospitals (rather than the secondary or primary level care Outpatient Clinics and Ambulatory/Day Treatment Centers) with the understanding they will receive better care, even before they know what their medical condition actually is! Further, the more individuals want to go the tertiary level care, rather than primary or secondary care levels actually drives up the cost of services for those who receive care, as many involve additional tests and procedures to "rule out" potential causes as the "duty of care" for Specialists is greater. Then, when the patients receive their bills for services rendered, they grumble and complain about the high cost of healthcare.

So, as Administrators, promote, support, and participate in education of the public and encourage proper use of the healthcare system when accessing services, as it reduces costs, waiting times, and making the secondary and tertiary care facilities available for the appropriate cases.

5. Always work to **have a good, friendly professional working relationship with your "competitor" healthcare facilities**, because in times of emergencies they can be your "best friends", and you, theirs.

This is an interesting set of circumstances, and is worthwhile to take initiatives to develop a good working relationship with Senior Management of both affiliated and "competition" hospitals and healthcare facilities. There will be time when your competitors can become your "best friends" in times of emergencies and the entire facility is at risk of being closed, or times when your facility may need a specific piece of equipment, either you transport your patient to their facility, or transport the necessary piece(s) of equipment to your facility. In either situation, you can develop a symbiotic relationship with your competitor. Here are two good examples of that type arrangement working.

The first was the situation where a maternity hospital was moving from an old facility to a new location, and there were many babies in ICU who needed to be transported from one location to the next, and the hospital did not have sufficient mobile incubators to effect the transfer, so arrangements were made with a nearby "competitor" hospital to borrow additional incubators to safely transfer the neonates across with minimal inconveniences to the neonates.

Another example was a specific mutual arrangement to make use of a "competitors" laboratory to process, blood products, and analysis. The Agreement was to use our Facility's laboratory to service our patients during the day, while allowing our competitor to use the Facility during our "off hours". As this was a mutual/reciprocal agreement, we would also have had access to their facility at night for our processing should the need occur. Fortunately, neither we nor our Competitor needed to activate the arrangement; however, it gave all "comfort" knowing we had alternative plans in place. This practice is also part of a good Business Continuity Plan.

6   It is **"relatively easy" to build hospitals** (i.e. bricks and mortar aspect), but often most **difficult to obtain the correct patient mix, necessary quantity of qualified manpower resources** required to operate the facility, i.e., Doctors/Specialists, Nurses, Technicians, Allied Health, and Administrators, etc.

On many occasions, we have been contacted by Developers, Businessmen and Investors who may be planning a new housing or business development. They project a community, new or old, will have a certain population and believe it to be a good corporate and social opportunity to have a hospital built to look after the community's medical needs besides potentially generating additional business.

While their intentions may be honorable, we counsel them that the building of the physical structure is the "relatively easy" part of a Hospital Project. In the overall planning, they should have a proper and complete Feasibility Study performed which takes into consideration many variables that can affect the success of the project. This step is "cheap insurance" to protect the potential investment. There will be major hurdles to overcome such as ability to recruit sufficient numbers of Specialist doctors, offering required Medical and Surgical Clinical specialties the community requires, and Nurses at various levels and with the necessary skillsets to support both the medical staff, as well as, operate the wards and services according to hospital required standards. Other professionals such as Pharmacists,

Imaging, Laboratory, and Therapist will also need to be engaged. Additionally, Hospital Administration professional staff with hospital or relevant healthcare background will be required to ensure all the components come together. Along with this, will be requirement to have access to sufficient financial strength to carry the Project through until such a point it will be operationally viable. This may take up to six years! This is the difficult part of the project, not the building of the structure. Remember building a hospital is one of the most complex business entities that can be built, which is heavily reliant on access to required manpower. Doctors and Nurses are always in short supply on an international basis, with very few countries producing enough medical and nursing professionals to cover their needs. So the only way to obtain the required medical staff will be to recruit from either the Public sector, which is normally one of the primary sources for recruitment, or encourage staff from existing facilities to change locations and affiliations that have been nurtured and developed over the years, by offering better "tools", locations, or opportunities to attract the Specialists. Not always so easy! This practice has the effect of creating a short term escalation spiral on salaries (until an equilibrium is once again achieved) so this practice must be carefully planned. If serious enough, feedback will be generated and efforts will be taken to seek a moratorium on "poaching" of staff of surrounding hospitals, so be aware and careful on how it is managed.

7   We must convince Developers and Planners to **build healthcare facilities** (hospitals, ambulatory care, clinics, etc.), **for long term operational efficiency**, and not just short term construction profit which

is all too often the situation. Invest a bit more up-front, as the initial investment becomes fixed and is depreciated over 40-50 years, otherwise the Operators/Owners will pay out increased operational expenses over the next 40-50 years, and the costs will be passed on to your patients/customers!

This is a difficult concept to have Developers accept. Right from the very start Developers typically set a budget for the construction and equipment of the facility, then try to make everything fit within the budget. This is typically "putting the cart before the horse" approach to planning. The proper approach should be to perform a proper Feasibility Study, identify the population to be served using the demographics of the area, and currently existing medical disciplines offered which then determines the medical specialties to be offered and the number of beds to be supported based on the number of Specialists who will commit to the facility. Once the basic medical service are agreed upon, then comes the design, construction and equipment planning phases specifying and selecting materials to allow for long term operational efficiency. Finally the financial requirements are determined, and discussed, and a strategy for equity and loans can be determined. Developers need to look at design and materials that offer lowest maintenance requirements over the next 40-50 years and define the requirements into the specifications, otherwise it will result in a facility requiring more frequent maintenance, higher utility bills that cost will be passed along to the patients in their bills. A good example I always use is the concept of installing "double glazed" windows, as well as double walls in the entire building, or in the worst case, the walls facing the sun, regardless of whether the facility is located in the temperate or tropical climate, particularly where air conditioning is used in all or part of the facility. The physics are the same, whether the preferred temperature on the inside is opposite the external ambient temperature. With double layer windows/walls, heat or cold preservation will be substantially improved, and will result in lower energy bills over the years. Another example is to structurally design the building so additional levels can be added in the future, and by installing wiring, ducting, medical gas piping, etc., up to any area that could be converted into ward, or clinical offices in the future. The Planners and Developers will only have one chance to build it correctly, and have the costs become part of the "sunk construction costs", depreciated over the life of the building, otherwise costs will be substantially higher in the future.

8   Keep an open mind as healthcare innovations in underdeveloped or developing countries have **many interesting and unique solutions to address issues,** both in processes and software. Be willing to observe, learn, and adapt.

We are all guilty of taking a position that only products or services from developed countries can meet and satisfy operational issues in under-developed or developing countries. This is an incorrect perception, and there are many times solutions have been developed, often time simple ones to address process flows and generating outcomes that meet or satisfy more sophisticated applications. Therefore, we should be willing to visit other countries, visit and tour local hospitals and healthcare facilities, observe operations, and software used to manage the business, ask questions, learn how they manage issues that are common to all, e.g., appointment scheduling, waiting time, order entry, results reporting, bill payment processing, and account settlement, etc., inspect and objectively determine if they are achieving the results being proposed, albeit using alternative methods (some may be rather basic or crude by developed standards and expectations). However, there may also be opportunities to learn new ways to operate the business. Basically, be "open minded" and willing to accept there may be new approaches, and help chart a path to greater and improved healthcare over a period of time.

9   When **purchasing medical equipment and surgical instruments, always obtain the items from reputable manufactures and sources**; otherwise, inexpensive items purchased will fail, could cause a negative outcome, resulting in legal action/exposure, while still needing to be replaced with quality equipment and instruments, thus incurring substantially more costs than a proper selection and investment up-front!

There is an old saying, "you get what you pay for", and that is particularly true when purchasing medical instruments, equipment, supplies and consumables. As a result we have always tried to obtain the best value for money, by being very detailed with our specifications, and ultimately securing items from reputable companies. There are many reasons for selecting the best items, even if they are not the least expensive, specifically, quality of material, design and construction, reliability, maintainability, and standards. Products with these attributes provide "value for money" as they maximize the "mean time between failures". Over the years, there have been instances where Doctors and Purchasing staff have tried to minimize expenses by solely focusing on cost of the items without sufficient consideration for the construction, material content, maintenance requirement, reliability, patient treatment, and legal aspects of utilizing inferior (and/or less expensive) items. One specific example was the selection of OR/OT instruments. Over objections, guidance, and advice based on years of experience from both myself and Director of Nursing, the Tender Selection and Evaluation Work Group Specialists selected a "package" of instruments to be used in the OR/OT from a non-traditional source due to a much lower price. After about three to six months of use, the instruments began failing, the first signs emerging as loss of their sharpened edges, and screws coming loose. A bit longer, we started obtaining feedback that the instrument metal was rusting, and failing during operations, with more than one surgeon becoming frustrated with the quality of the instruments (literally throwing them across the OR/OT, and verbally expressing their unhappiness on the OR/OT Nurses), and demanding administration purchase better replacement instrument or they will not perform their surgeries at the hospital. Fortunately, there were no operations whose outcomes were negatively affected (to our knowledge) as a result of any inter-operative instrument failures. Had there been an incident, both the hospital and surgeons could have been subjected to a medical malpractice suit, resulting in expensive legal proceedings, settlements, negative media and loss of credibility.

To the credit of the surgeons, once the problems started to arise, the surgeons on the subsequent Tender Selection and Evaluation Work Group took guidance and advice from both myself and my Nursing Director to prepare the necessary specification list, and inviting only pre-qualified reputable companies, who provided selected samples of their instruments for evaluation, allowing the Evaluation Work Group to make a selection from one or more companies. Once the replacements were acquired and put into service, all the complaints, and problems previously experienced, were resolved. However, this came at a cost to the hospital; they spent money for the initial instrument investment, and then had to re-invest in another set of high quality replacements which were from reputable companies, so the "cheap" instruments were a complete "write-off".

This same situation was experienced when selecting other medical equipment, e.g., 3D echo machine, monitors, beds, etc. used throughout the hospital, supplies, consumables, and pharmaceuticals (patented, vs generic). Cost must be balanced with quality.

Often, items are selected exclusively based on price, not on quality, or documented incidents from staff or patients. Patients trust the doctors, hospital and staff with their lives, so staff have an obligation to take the necessary steps to protect and ensure patients receive the best treatment possible, using proven, reliable products.

I close with the old adage, "do not be penny wise and pound foolish"!

10   **Healthcare is one of three industries that will always be relevant.** People will need medical services throughout their life, people need to eat, and people will pass away. This also allows the industry

to survive recession cycles with minimal impact compared to other industries, with softened ups and downs, but in a general, an upward trend over time.

The lifelong need for food, and final arrangements for our passing are well recognized; however, we wish to draw attention for the lifelong need and requirement of healthcare services.

Healthcare, in most countries, actually starts before birth, with observation and follow-up on the mother's progress during pregnancy, and proactive planning for a successful delivery. After birth, babies need attention, to be protected from diseases that affect or afflict babies, and toddlers as they journey through their early years and become exposed to and develop immunities to the germs that abound in the environment. In most instances children will become ill, but in that process become stronger, and are able to combat repeated exposure. Where their natural and acquired immunities fail, it may result in them having to be treated either as outpatients, or if necessary, as inpatients.

Likewise, as children mature and become young adults and adults they will require medical and surgical care due to accidents, trauma, infection, pregnancies both as outpatients and inpatients. As they grow older, other age related conditions and complications will arise requiring chronic treatments and/or acute interventions. Support services, medications, and use of physical aides, ranging from spectacles, hearing aids, pace makers, dental, implants, and rehabilitation will be required as they recover from various illnesses and conditions, up until the time they require palliative care and comfort in their final hours. The point being made is that throughout one's life, the need and seeking of healthcare will be required.

Illnesses do not follow economic cycles (but they may have their own cycles), so healthcare will be required based on the severity of the condition that emerges and resources available. While there will be times immediate treatment can be deferred for a period of time, normally at some point it will become "urgent" and need to be addressed, lest it become more critical with emerging co-morbidities and complications that could result in fatal outcomes. What pattern that does emerge during economic downturns, is for patients and families to shift more to outpatient, day care/ambulatory care treatments services, and if admission to a hospital is necessary, to seriously consider and explore lower cost options (e.g. medical management vs surgical intervention; traditional treatments vs "cutting edge" procedures; Government vs Private hospital), or selections of a lower Class of services with greater subsidy (government support) or less spacious accommodations. However, as cost of manpower in healthcare will increase over time due to inflation, there will be peaks, and with economic downturns/recessions there will be valleys that will require healthcare delivery systems to conserve and rationalize dwindling funding/revenue resources, while internally exploring new processes, and developing creative new techniques to contain or reduce costs while moving into a new cycle.

Remember, while the healthcare industry will experience economic peaks and valleys, they are normally not as severe or massive in swings as manufacturing and many other service related industry cycles, e.g. hotel, tourist, and if managed and planned carefully, with cooperation of the staff, basic services can be preserved to treat patients.

11 **Healthcare is a fascinating industry as the "landscape" is constantly changing.** New technologies are always being developed, new procedures identified with good clinical outcomes, new equipment designed, new discoveries in medical science to improve life management, and treatment. For all these reasons, healthcare is one of the most exciting industries to be affiliated.

While change is a constant in all industry sectors, the pace of change in healthcare is one of the fastest. Funding, research, Information Technology (IT), robotics, artificial intelligence (AI), changing demographic profiles (aging baby boomers), military battlefield requirements, shortage of professional staff (especially doctors, specialists, nurses) all exert pressures on healthcare systems to streamline service delivery while improving survival outcomes. For all those reasons, and more, this makes healthcare a dynamic, interesting, and challenging industry in which to be involved. The healthcare industry includes not only all clinics, hospitals, but the entire continuum of care spectrum, from primary services to end of life; as well as the pharmaceutical (drugs, medications), allied health/clinical support (laboratories, pharmacy, imaging, therapies, etc.), Information Technology related, e.g. digitized medical records, robotics, artificial intelligence (AI) etc., Bio-Medical service providers, along with all the operational, facility, and administrative support services, supply chain and consumable management, medical equipment companies, prosthetics that complement the clinical components.

With all of these dimensions independently, and collectively operating at various stages of maturity, this creates unique opportunities for individuals and companies to grow and develop new products, and services in healthcare, making the healthcare an industry in which one can be proud to be associated.

12   Life as a **Chief, Director, or Senior Manager** is challenging.

Listed below is a "litany of responsibilities" for individuals in the various Chief positions (or their equivalents), Directors and Senior Managers which highlights a number of key expectations. It is exciting, as well as demanding, and requires selection of individuals who have both commitment and the necessary strength to meet the expectations.

12.1   Living a life of "greys". By the time issues or problems reach you, they are not the easy "black and white" situations. Often, you need to take a decision with the best, but limited information,

12.2   Needing to identify, learn, and understand "**basic/ first principles**" as they become your "guiding light" as you take decisions, or make recommendations,

12.3   Being the first level to translate "intent and strategy" into operational, and defined objectives,

12.4   Keeping open lines of communications to peers, bosses, subordinates, or others you respect in the field to obtain reliable information to assist you in understanding a problem,

12.5   Accepting you are always "on call", even when you are not "on call",

12.6 Defending the organization, and all its people.... they are your people,
12.7 Being a communicator, resolver, and solver,
12.8 Being humble and never forgetting your origins. The same people who supported your growth and development can also affect your future,
12.9 Being prepared to take on challenges, for which you were never trained,
12.10 Learning to delegate where appropriate,
12.11 Developing the next level,
12.12 Not micro-managing because if this is necessary, you have the wrong individuals as Managers,
12.13 Being prepared to take risk,
12.14 Not every decision you take will be the correct one, but you **should** make more correct ones than incorrect,
12.15 You may need to make many decisions with less than 60% of the information, but will be held 100% accountable,
12.16 By the time you get 100% of the information, you become redundant,
12.17 Being prepared to be criticized as you have become a "target" and "official representative" of the organization,
12.18 Being a "cheerleader",
12.19 Having long days,
12.20 Never being paid for "overtime",
12.21 Recognizing that the reward for performing "above average" means continued employment,
12.22 Being professional at all times,

12.23 Recognizing that whatever you say, or do reflects on the organization,

12.24 Knowing there are never any "off the record" comments,

12.25 Being looked upon as a leader, and taking action as required,

12.26 Being challenged and "loving it"!

12.27 **Most REWARDING......!!!**

Those identified will be given responsibilities, and training as part of the grooming process for succession planning. Over the course of development, many will fail to meet the requirements due to various internal and external commitments such as, family pressure (raising a family, family/relative bias toward healthcare, marital issues), psychological (stress management, managing outbreak crisis), general health, or other emerging constraints, as the demands are substantial. However, for the ones who succeed in managing the expectations, they can ultimately "retire" knowing they have made a contribution to the organization and their profession while mentoring and developing future administrators.

13   **P&Ps are designed to cover about 95% of all situations and processes** encountered in an organization. Management and Administrators contribute by addressing the remaining 5% of the situations.

As part of good corporate governance, Policies and Procedures (P&Ps) also known at Standard Operating Procedures (SOPs) are developed into a set of documents that capture various company policies (position statements) and identifying practices/procedures, which are followed in proper sequence, to achieve expected results. They are normally Department specific in terms of ownership, management compliance, and responsibility, yet may require compliance from a few to many other Departments, so they must be coordinated and integrated. High level Company/Corporate wide P&Ps are applicable to all Departments. Many P&Ps are general in nature, while certain ones are specific in scope and application. Clinical and direct hands-on types of P&Ps must be in place with mandatory compliance required by staff at opening of a facility. Most P&Ps are evolving, to be reviewed, refined and regularly updated to capture changes (major and minor) in processes and procedures so they are kept current. These documents establish the "intent baselines and principles" when taking actions for most activities, and indexed accordingly. Should any situations arise where outcomes differ from the P&Ps intent, compliance (or non-compliance) with the approved P&Ps can have legal implications, either to protect the staff and organization against legal challenges if they were followed, or to establish liability if they were not followed, or were flawed.

Properly developed P&Ps provide clear guidelines for most activities, estimated at about 95%; however, there are legitimate situations that fail to fit into the prescribed sequences, and require Supervisors, Managers, and Senior Management in the hierarchy to make an interpretation. Even they must take decisions based on their professional understanding of "principles, intent, and spirit", of the P&P to resolve, and keep the organization in good operation. Final decisions can go in either direction, but all the decision takers must assume responsibility for the outcomes of their interpretations and implementation. Where possible, we try to give the "benefit of doubt" to the individual(s) raising the issues where guidelines points may be ambiguous, yet not contravene any serious principles. This action both "closes" the immediate issue, and treats the associated activities as a "learning point", and provides an opportunity to make whatever changes to the existing policies to preclude repeat of the situation. This is where the Administrators and Management earn their salary. Related to this many individuals often comment on the salaries of Management, but when asked if they would be prepared to take decisions under similar circumstances knowing the associated potential responsibilities, most will decline the opportunity.

14   Remember to **treat your strategic "business partners" as your own staff**. Outsourcing is a management tool, and staff providing services under this arrangement should be treated, and included, as if they were on payroll.

Healthcare delivery is the primary objective of a hospital or healthcare facility (clinic(s), ambulatory service, etc.). Apart from certain administration roles, management has the prerogative to outsource many other "non-core" services to external companies who specialize in the services required, and offer staff career paths that would be limited or nonexistent in the stand alone hospital or healthcare facility environment. The outsourcing model often offers a cost effective solution as well, for provision of the needed service. "Business Partner" arrangements are normally administered by contracts stipulating what services are to be provided (i.e., deliverables), and various metrics for measuring compliance, just as those that would be in effect if the Department were staffed with in-house (payroll staff) positions. Outsourcing partners are common for many facility support services, such as housekeeping/environmental; catering/food service (kitchen); facility engineering and maintenance, bio-medical engineering, landscaping and grounds keeping; waste collection and removal; patient transport; ambulance; and security etc. Certain administrative support services also lend themselves to outsourcing such as Accounts Receivable; Debt Collections; Accounting; Legal Services; Human Resources/Personnel; Marketing/Advertising; Public Relations; Corporate Communications; etc.

Management, Finance and Human Resource must recognize the staff who are assigned to the hospital or healthcare facility as part of the Business Partner affiliation, they must be treated as if they were staff on the hospital or healthcare facility's direct payroll! Given the relationship, the number of Full Time Equivalent (FTEs) the Business Partner employs must also be reported to both HR and Finance for inclusion in the total FTE count of the organization, i.e. employed (directly or indirectly) for reporting and comparison purposes. NOTE: It is a common practice for HR/Personnel, and Finance/Accounting Departments in failing to recognize these FTE numbers since they are "not on payroll", which understates the total manpower utilized in delivery of services and affects the accuracy of comparative data when comparing similar organizations, and does not give the "full picture" of FTEs engaged and match against the approved numbers.

The Business Partners and their staff should be informed of any conditions relating to their health and welfare within the organization. Further, as they are part of the hospital or healthcare facility, their efforts and contributions should be recognized just as payroll staff. A good example was the SARs outbreak. Once the outbreak was under control, various organizations initiated distribution of books and small financial tokens to reward the staff on payroll only. However, Management took the initiative to also provide a "small token" to our Business Partners as well, so their staff could also be recognized. This was appreciated by the Business Partners and made their staff more dedicated. Whenever there is a potential outbreak situation, N-95 masks and thermometers may be provided to payroll staff, but provision should also be made to supply the Business Partner staff with the same items. They are part of the "facility family" and faced the same, and sometimes worse working conditions! Treat them fairly and as family.

The point is, a Board approves a specific number of Full Time Equivalent (FTE) positions in the annual budget, and hospital or healthcare management normally has operational authority and flexibility to fill various positions as either direct hires or as part of a Business Partner solution. So, those staff should be considered as an extension of the payroll staff and FTEs counted. Consider, if all administrative services (Finance, HR) and support services (Labs, Imaging, Pharmacy, Rehab) were outsourced, does that mean no staff are required to provide services? This thinking is neither rational nor reasonable, so include them.

15. What **employment as a healthcare professional means**. If you are hired/paid part time, you will work full time; when you hired/paid full time, you

work up to double time ++! It is known as "value for money".

An interesting phenomenon in healthcare is that an individual (in a professional Supervisor or Manager Level position and above, all the way to the top) never work a normal defined week schedule for any length of time. Due to deadlines, audits, workload, meetings at all hours of the day and week, attendances at seminars and conferences, drafting or writing Senior Management or Board Level papers, reading other reports, drafts for comment or approval, authorizing payments, etc., you generally cannot complete all those tasks within the confines of a normal workweek. At these levels, work may be conducted in the prescribed office, but is not restricted to the confines of the office, so often work is "brought home" to finish either "on line with the office computers" or on a company laptop. Often we complete reading necessary documents, and making both local and international telephone calls either after returning home, whatever time that is, to whatever hours in the early morning, i.e. midnight plus, and over the weekends as required in order to meet various schedules or deadlines. While you try to arrive at work at the prescribed time, normally between the hours of 8 to 9 am, (sometimes earlier as required) in order to manage, meet, distribute, delegate, supervise, consult about other activities involving others, staff counseling, etc., so completing all the tasks and duties required normally fall short of the available hours in the day. During all my years at work, and individuals I have had the privilege to worked with, all typically will "clock" up to 60-80++ hours per week addressing all the tasks, both at work, and various other locations we may need to visit. Travel for meetings at other locations further expands the hours dedicated to work related activities. Hence the observation that senior staff can work up to twice the normal hours.

When we take on appointments/assignments on a "part time" basis, we have always ensured the company has received the scheduled hours per the agreement but also included hours up to twice the initial commitment. So a commitment of half time often results in work equivalent approaching a full time appointment.

In both instances I have never heard professional, dedicated healthcare individuals complain because most individual in healthcare accept the time commitment as part of the expectations to perform, and a contribution to keeps the organization functioning. The ones who cannot manage the commitment normally leave healthcare for other professions or industries. So all this time invested is reflected as "value for money" in terms our commitment to the industry and professions. If it goes above those levels, the organization must seriously consider hiring additional staff!

16   When negotiating Contractual Terms, always view the Terms from the perspective that you could be engaged (hired or assigned) in the future to manage the Contract, by the other Party! **Would you be satisfied with them and consider them reasonable and balanced.**

Negotiating "terms of agreement" for a contract can be quite detailed and exasperating at times. When developing the contract/agreement document, both parties need to agree on the scope, metrics, and expectations to be achieved, as well as, inclusion of various clauses to address any breaches that may occur and the remedies available. In that process the document design should be balanced and fair to both parties. In various situations, the "other party" may already have a draft document they are using, or have used in other Agreements, and offer to use it to expedite the signing process; however, always read the document to ensure the terms are balanced. It is interesting that in many instances the terms are very biased towards protecting the interests of one side, the "other party", to the detriment of your organization, so this must be addressed and remedied during the negotiation phase. I have also experienced a situation where I was involved in negotiating terms for an Agreement, and then "by fate" some years later I joined the "other party" of the Agreement and it became my responsibility to manage the Contract based on the terms developed earlier. Fortunately, the terms were reasonable, so it was relatively easy to understand, comply, and administer. Had the Agreement not been balanced, it would have been most difficult to assume the role.

So the message to be learned is to be "balanced and fair" in the negotiations, learn the key objectives of the organization with whom you are contracting, and make an effort to design the Agreement in a manner you would be satisfied with, if you switched sides.

17   The difference between a CFO/FC and other junior Finance/Accounting positions, (or any other senior position professionals in the organization), is that they have learned to look at the organization and all its operations **HOLISTICALLY, as they must "see**

and appreciate the big picture" and take decisions accordingly.

Many times during my career, I have been asked "what is the difference between being a Chief Financial Officer or Finance Controller", and other finance and accounting positions. Is it not just a higher level position with similar responsibilities and expectations but greater recognition? Similar questions have been raised about other Senior Management positions i.e. CEO, COO, Chairman Medical Board, Chief Nursing Officer, or their equivalents and my response has always been it is about the individual's ability to "see the big picture" of the organization. One may be or have been very good as the Head of a Department, Division, or in a number two position, but that does not ensure they will perform well in the most senior of positions. At the higher level, one needs to overcome individual biases and preferences based on one's background and look Holistically to what is best for the organization, to strengthen areas of weakness, look for growth opportunities, or be critical and able to "downsize" if necessary, refocus in certain areas, question everything being done, or "get back to basics" for the company's survival and growth. One must be neutral and work well with all parties to achieve Board objectives.

The CFO is no longer the low level "number cruncher", where one is tracking the small dollar and cents (or equivalents), but rather looking at numbers rounded off to the thousands or millions to determine if actions, proposals, and outcomes are correct. CFOs require an understanding of financial structuring or how to manage an IPO, legal terms, regulatory requirements of various Government Ministries/Departments, IT areas, and reinforced with exposure to as many revenue generating operational Departmental services. If an individual has yet to mature to that level and assumes the role of CFO while still personally delving into minutia of daily operations (their comfort zone), they will ultimately fail, as they will miss what is happening at higher levels, both within the organization, with competition, and in the regional or international environment. To manage internal workings one should use the chain of command to ensure operations are being performed correctly by having regular (daily, weekly, monthly) update meetings from Division/Department Heads either on a one-to-one basis or in a structured management meeting. Internal Auditors or External Consultants can be directed to observe and analyze questionable actions or areas of concern to provide objective feedback, and raise issues and points for rectification or improvement. Management Points from external auditors also provide feedback on the internal status of operations.

So, for CFO or any other senior management position, having a Holistic perspective is critical. If the CFO has evolved with a healthcare background, it is easier for them to assume the position; however, financial professionals from other industries can be "oriented and trained", preferably under the "mentorship" of an experienced healthcare financial professional. Other senior management professionals should also be guided by Mentors if possible.

18 Observation. Best **time for Meetings with Doctors/ Specialists** is usually early in the morning, before rounds and/or starting clinics/surgical sessions, sometime around lunch time, or late in the afternoon after completion of their clinical duties, but

definitely not in the middle of the their session times. Provision of food makes the Meetings more appreciated.

At times there are legitimate reasons to meet up with the Medical staff relating to issues both administrative and clinical in nature, where their input and recommendations is required. In those instances, the administrative staff will typically be tasked with making necessary arrangements and locating a venue. I have had to manage the perceptions of the staff, both administrative and operational who express frustrations in their efforts to arrange for meetings with the doctors, nurses, or other clinical staff. Unless it is an emergency situation, such as responding to an outbreak of some sort or a major threat, we need to be sensitive about holding meetings during the prime times during the day during scheduled morning rounds, consultation, or operation/treatment hours. We have found the best time to meet up with the Doctors/Specialists in particular, is in the early morning hours before start of their daily rounds, during scheduled lunchtime providing food, or late afternoon, or after hours, typically six pm or later. Again, offering of food is appreciated and makes the meeting go smoother. So in these instances, the administrative staff need to be prepared to arrive early in the morning or stay after normal Clinical work hours, sometimes both in the same day, as it may be difficult for all the medical staff to be available at one time.

The primary message is to be considerate of Doctors time and their commitment to treating patients, so arrange meetings with Medical staff at times that avoid conflicting with their normal, scheduled practice hours. Keep in mind, if patient appointments are already set for the day, any delay attending to the first patient of morning will have a "knock-on" effect of delaying attendances of all subsequent patients appointments in the session (normally four hours), which may result in unnecessary complaints over extended waiting time and will add to the stress of the nurses managing the Clinics or Operating Rooms/Theatres.

19 When introducing new programs or processes, **make sure you take time to know and understand the current ones and their linkages**, to avoid blindly updating one component while affecting or disrupting other features or backroom support functions.

Problems will always occur, and solutions will need to be found; however, we must exercise caution, and perform "what I call" a 360° review on all other systems that might "touch upon" the changes being made to determine we do not introduce new problems which will take longer to untangle and correct in the future. This concept is applicable both in the computer programming "fixes", as well as process, and operational changes. A simple example of where problems may arise is when fixing computer related problems. Consider where code is written to accept "variable" input by the End User which can change the output results, e.g. simple "$x + y = x$" equation. However, when trying to rectify a problem, unbeknownst to the End User, the simple equation was modified (for some reason) with a hard coded fixed number(s) which are taken into consideration by the computer, so obviously the results will be impacted the inclusion of the hardcoded number, e.g. "$x+y+2.55 = x$". The "hard coded" component which does not change with the variable data, will impact the outcome of the expected results. Rather than a number, it could be text, symbols, linkages, "what ifs" which could have the same impact, and give an incorrect answer.

So, when changes to computer Code are made, an individual MUST be tasked to review ALL the lines of Code to determine if any other modifying factor is present. Further, sufficient computer generated outcomes should be compared to manually calculated outcomes, to validate the changes are working properly before "sign-off" acceptance.

20 **Doctors/Specialists must be appointed to lead and drive clinically related accreditation/certification related initiatives**, e.g. JCI, FACT, ISO, etc., who can engage and mobilize the entire organization. "Non-clinician" led initiatives will fail to achieve the same level of commitment and "buy-in", as it will be merely perceived as another administrative requirement rather than for clinical benefit.

Whenever a clinically related decision needs to be taken affecting accreditation or other related certification processes within the organization, it is imperative that at least one clinician perceives the benefit of all the time and effort to adopt the initiative and then becomes a clinical "champion". This acceptance must be driven by a clinician; otherwise, it will be perceived as another administrative task to be implemented, without the conviction to make the initiative work. For Joint Commission International (JCI), there are many auditable guidelines that must be addressed in detail and demonstrated by documentation for a defined minimum period of time to achieve a successful accreditation.

A majority of the guidelines relate to acceptable medical/clinical care standards and "best" practices, as well as a number of operational and construction practices, so participation and "buy-in" from the Clinicians is critical. Without a core of specialists appreciating the potential clinical benefits both in terms of local and international recognition and reputation, as well as the financial benefits attributable to operating in a hospital meeting the JCI standards (or equivalent) the investment in time and resources will be lost, both of which are substantial.

Efforts of non-clinicians in leading the initiative will often fail to achieve the same level of commitment, engagement or enthusiasm, as it will be perceived as just another "administrative exercise" that detracts from the clinician's primary mission of treating patients. Only once the organization makes the effort and ultimately achieves accreditation, can they place the official logo on their letterhead, and business cards, do they really appreciate the efforts made. So we want to encourage all Clinicians to take up the challenges to have their Hospitals and facilities seek national or international recognition through accreditation from respected and reputable certification entities.

21   A good **clinical or administrative initiative presented before its time will fail to gather support**. Both the infrastructure (staff, technology) and mindset must be ready for the change to occur.

Many ideas or concepts, after initial filtering, will surface and be worth consideration, presentation and discussion within the organization. An observation made over the years is that if an organization has yet to mature or taken strategic decisions about future positioning, then any concepts or related ideas will be downplayed with various reasons or justifications for deferring the proposal being introduced. A simple example was a concept of introducing Joint Commission, International (JCI) Accreditation into a hospital as this was considered the international healthcare "gold standard" by which to measure clinical and operational performance. As no other Hospital in the region had adopted the concept, the clinical view was that the demanding requirements were not relevant (at that time) in the local environment, so the proposal was shelved. About two or three years later, one of the well-known facilities in the region adopted the concept, implemented the program, and achieved accreditation. This opened opportunities for all the Hospital to broaden their International Service base, and become Referral Centers for patients from as far away as the United States (patients wishing for a medical holiday, or for expats living in Asian countries needing medical care), since with the JCI accreditation, patients/hospital were able to access US based insurance companies for partial or complete reimbursement which made seeking medical services in Singapore, Bangkok and the Region affordable and convenient. Given the success and recognition achieved, all the hospitals in the Region accepted the idea, and ultimately adopted the JCI Accreditation Standards. A good example of an "idea before its time" yet required an external event to give the proposal the needed rationale for implementation. Similar examples can also be observed for implementation of various integrated software (Pharmacy,

Laboratory, Imaging, Supply Management, Operating Room/ Theatre systems), that facilitated in more coordinated clinical management (results reporting, DRGs, and disease tracking) as well as concurrent capture of the services performed and timely billing of services to patients with a view of having a bill ready to the patient at or shortly after the point of discharge. Additional ideas that have yet to gain general acceptance are related to more efficient building construction to reduce energy consumption e.g., double glazed windows and reduce repairs, implementation of Enterprise Risk Management (ERM) and Business Continuity Planning (BCP), senior villages, etc.

Note, JCI is an international accrediting agency that helps achieve best standards, and best practices in delivery of healthcare in Hospitals, Freestanding Ambulatory Centers, and Outpatient Specialty Clinics. So, by achieving JCI accreditation the Institutions enjoy both the standards benefit as well as the insurance benefit if interested. However, new country specific "accreditation standards" are being developed which meet local needs, may be taken into consideration. The important principle is to develop and adopt clinical standards that can be universal, measurable, and sustainable.

22   One must recognize that in every system **there are solutions to various situations which** would allow for more cost effective use of limited resources yet still achieve satisfactory outcomes, but **cannot be adopted for sensitive, internal or external, political or policy reasons.**

This is sensitive topic that must be recognized and managed properly without creating negative perceptions on high level decisions without understanding the principles involved when certain policy decisions are taken.

The Corporate Board or Directors/Trustees, Ministry/Department of Health or Finance level entities often take decisions based on political commitments, or other special considerations for the benefit of the entire population, which may not always appear consistent with normal, good business practices, yet they serve an important role in healthcare delivery so we need to accept them, pending any change in the governmental directions but with a view they will be reviewed periodically.

This results in situations where charges for certain services are not all in alignment with approved pricing policy formulae, for patients meeting certain admission criteria (private/subsidized, age or medical condition stratified), pre-approval for referral from specific charitable organizations where charges may be automatically reduced or waived. Rationalizing of limited resources and access by patients resulting in extended waiting times ranging from weeks, months, or even years. Normally when this occurs, the amounts reduced or absorbed are accumulated (by Accounting Department) and reported to specific departments responsible for monitoring utilization, ensuring pricing policies which support specific target groups are implemented and to validate amounts of funding provided. The reason this is mentioned is because staff, patients, or others not familiar with the history, will ask "why" this process or service fails to align with stated practices or questions the amenities of services provided. We need to explain there are exceptions and other consideration or principles that need to be satisfied to rationalize services within the organization or country for which we provide services.

Any deviations that conflict with policy, or ethics of the organization, can and often will affect operational procedures, and require "work around" alternative solutions as they are exceptions to the normal rules. Several good examples of the situation is where charges are "capped" either by government, compliance with national insurance schemes, contracts with private insurance companies, special pricing of services for defined groupings/classes of patients particularly where government funding/subvention or grants are involved. Alternatively, certain procedures are charged at full price, rather than being eligible for partial or complete funding by government, or insurance scheme. There are reasons, and when the topics are periodically raised, explanations are provided, and we are directed to comply with the guidelines, but we should take time to learn and understand the variations so staff can respond in an intelligent manner. It is important, from an operational level to comply with the Board/Trustees, Ministry/Department of Health/Finance or other higher levels that provide funding and instructions on expectations; however, we should periodically raise the topics for future review and consideration should there be changes in underlying technology, service expectations, perceptions on the way to manage, as well as changes in political or Board direction.

23   In times of economic downturns or serious cost containment/reduction/right sizing environment, **when manpower costs must be reduced, make**

sure there is a proper financial balance between professional and support staff. It is often the first reaction to reduce the number (FTE) of support staff (clerks, attendants, secretaries, technicians, facility engineers, etc.) who ensure the daily detailed operations and documentation are managed, to meet the FTE or dollar targets. Rather, **for a "first cut", take this as an opportunity to "cull" certain marginal/non-productive professional staff to save the junior staff.** Seasoned Managers take decisions accordingly. The approach also applies to junior staff.

All industries experience business cycles, some last a short time, others longer, some more severe, some milder, it is a reality. Certain cycles occur on relatively short notices, others have longer, more predictable cycles. Healthcare is no different, but in private hospitals the impact can be greater if they are servicing a higher patient mix from regional or international sources. Conversely, hospitals (private and government related) primarily serving the local population are less affected. The hospital cycles tend to follow the normal economic cycles but are usually less severe, as the population tends to require medical services, regardless of the economic cycle. Elective or non- critical procedures may be selectively deferred until the economy improves at private hospitals with patients shifting to government affiliated hospitals due to lower charges, but all emergency, urgent, and obstetric related cases continue to require treatment.

Depending on severity of the economic conditions, Management and the Board will require operations to adjust their expenses to minimize disruption of the core services defined and provided by the hospital/healthcare facility. The first area reviewed is normally the Capital Expense Budget (CAPEX) for equipment (replacement, new), renovation of existing facilities, or construction of new facilities, as well as new minimal or non-revenue generating related program expenses. After review, any CAPEX items that can be deferred will be.

Next will be the review of the Operating Expense Budget (OPEX). Normally 45-60+% of a hospital's total expenses are manpower related, so Finance will perform necessary calculations to determine revised Budget numbers based on input and assessment from the Senior Management and the Board. Given the high percentage of the OPEX Budget being manpower, it will be required to make a contribution in the OPEX Budget savings. Supplies, consumables, can contribute variably and fixed cost items contribute little to saving. (NOTE: In certain countries, due to high import taxes levied on drugs, medical supplies, and equipment, the cost of these items can actually constitute a larger component of operations than manpower, so Operation Management must review options available and select items, either local or imported, that best meet the Clinician's needs, and can be justified in terms of both improved patient management, and overall cost management).

So a serious manpower review should be performed. The first "wave" of review should be to focus on professional staff on payroll making marginal performance contributions in services for various reasons, such as, reducing workload (phasing down) as they are nearing planned retirement, having increased personal or family related medical issues requiring frequent leave requirements, generally low productivity level, and receiving "marginal" appraisals from their supervisors. While these staff provide incremental contributions, in times of serious economic downturn the organization must focus on retaining manpower who can perform at optimal levels.

A similar review would be in order for the support and administrative staff who also fit the same profile, so there is a balanced contribution towards manpower savings amongst all levels throughout the organization. If these efforts are still insufficient to satisfy the revised budget projections, then additional reviews of benefits, and services offered need to be examined, with emphasis on continued compliance with defined patient to staff ratios in core service/treatment areas, while potentially suspending non-core programs.

In many hospitals/healthcare facilities, management tends to limit their "field of vision" to junior grade staff, or those with low seniority for retrenchment and downsizing exercises to the detriment of the organization, as many of these individuals serve and support the professional staff, so with their reduction, it creates an excess burden on the remaining junior staff, as well as the professional staff.

Recognizing the need to maintain as many defined services within the hospital/healthcare facility operational at all times, another excellent, creative strategy has been implemented. In various hospitals and hospital groups, to preserve manpower during times of downturns or crisis, there is an agreement (with the Union and/or within individual employment contracts) for all staff to take voluntary/mandatory pay reductions of "x percent" to achieve the balance of the reduction required. This can be built into salary component as a "fixed" and a "variable" component, e.g., 90/10%, 85-15%. This organization wide contributory approach can actually achieve all or a great part of any required OPEX savings, while preserving productive staff to maintain services, and "sending a message" to all staff that they are important which helps improve morale during difficult times. Once the economic and workload conditions stabilize, and start to recover, the percentages reduced can be reinstated. This concept requires support from the highest levels, specifically Board level, and "buy-in" from all employee representation groups, which typically follow a "seniority" model to succeed.

24   Exceptional Managers **always ask WHY** for both good or bad outcomes, as well as looking for trends. This is the only way to learn and know the business.

A necessary personality trait of Managers and above must nurture is their motivation to understand what is happening and explore and learn as much as possible about any outcome, both good/positive and bad/negative. Why was it good or bad? It is this inquisitive nature that will facilitate Managers to learn and understand the product, or services, with which they are involved. At the same time Managers should always be looking at trends, and asking "why" for any performance above or below their expected targets. Based on the Manager's experience they should know if any actions need to be taken and the magnitude. If the direction is negative, then effort must be expended to learn the reason "why" and plan for corrective action. Conversely, if better than expected, they must review resources to determine if they are sufficient to support the increased workload.

So by monitoring workload and trends and managing the key elements affecting the performance, the Manager can take necessary actions early enough to make an impact. In the meantime, the Manager is getting to "know the business" and becoming more valuable in the process. Always explore and ask "WHY"!

25 **Organizations use Consultants for three primary reasons**:
25.1 Lack of skills, knowledge, time, or manpower to address opportunities,
25.2 Verification/validation of internally generated information,
25.3 Manage and implement difficult situations, e.g., downsizing/right sizing, restructuring, major reorganization.

Consultants serve an important role in complementing Senior Management of an organization. They are normally engaged for one of the three primary reasons indicated above for a limited period of time, to complete a specific set of deliverables according to the Scope of Works detailed in the engagement contract.

In most instances Consultants are specialized in specific areas and are individuals or companies who can perform high level strategic reviews and development, as well as detailed operational assessments within an organization to identify areas for improvement. Consultants are contracted to offer skills on a temporary basis for implementation of strategic initiatives, building designs, improving workflow and operational improvement processes, as well as introduction of industry best practices. Given the range of an organization's need, there may not be sufficient or correct staff with the necessary skillsets or experience to effect the desired changes, so the use of external Consultants offers the best option. For example, an organization may engage the "independent" Consulting Service of an Auditing Firm appointed to perform the annual financial audit, or Consulting Service of another large Accounting firm to provide recommendations on how to improve internal control, billing flow, collection process, or investment management in finance; or, an architectural firm to provide new designs and renderings for renovation, expansion, facility related energy saving plans. There are many other types of Consultants with skills ranging from strategic planning, operational workflow, IT infrastructure, purchasing, space planning, legal/contractual compliance, clinical practice "best practice", or introduction/implementation of clinical pathways to name a few.

Secondly, Consultants are often used for verification and validation purposes with the added potential of offering complementary ideas or services to implement changes that have been identified. Again organizations may have good ideas, but require feedback and a review of their ideas to determine if they are implementable. The Consultants may subject the proposed changes/ideas to Strength, Weakness, Opportunity, Threat (SWOT), Political, Economic, Social, Technical (PEST), Enterprise Risk Management (ERM) analysis, as well as perform a Feasibility and/or a Financial Study analysis to determine if the concepts or ideas are achievable, and then assist the organization in the correct implementation approach.

The third reason for use of Consultants is to engage an independent, third party (individual or company) to perform certain difficult tasks, not only because they have the necessary expertise, but also act as a buffer for the Board when implementing paradigm shifting ideas, such as a major government, financial, or organizational restructuring that would be too difficult or sensitive for existing management infrastructure to manage and execute. Consultants can also be engaged to manage down-sizing ("right-sizing) decisions, which may involve in release, replacement, or finding alternative employment (where appropriate) for specific individuals affected. The Consultants can be involved in developing various "exit" and "out-placement" packages to facilitate affected staff. At the end of the major exercise, and the Consultants have completed their tasks, the contract is completed, and the Consultants leave and become the "bad guys" who initiated the changes, leaving local management with less stress over the actions taken. NOTE: After the changes have been effected, they will most likely be maintained even if there are a few disgruntled and sometimes vocal individuals. However, over time, most will accept and adapt, or leave.

The key benefits in the use of Consultants is that the organization is gaining access to specific expertise for a limited and known time duration, and the costs can be planned and will end once the engagement is completed.

26   When you **work as a Consultant to a healthcare organization, your observations, recommendations are seriously accepted and acted upon.** If you "join" the organization, new

ideas and recommendations are treated as normal, expected contributions from staff, and a new set of Consultants are engaged!

This is an interesting anomaly that both I and others have personally experienced, or have expressed similar observations.

Whenever external Consultants, Auditors or other independent professionals are engaged to perform specific services, projects, assessments, or assignments, the resulting recommendation(s) are usually eagerly anticipated by Management or Board who normally accept and adopt the recommendation in total or with minimal modifications. Given the substantial amounts of money paid, this is a good outcome and expectation by both parties.

But I have both participated in and observed others who have taken the step to transition from independent external Consultant to join the organization at the request of Management (providing there are no exclusion clauses prohibiting engagement of their staff for specific period of time, normally ranging from six months to three years, depending on the industry and technology levels involved). Initially, the individuals are still valued as "special project" individuals for three to six months and most recommendations from the assigned "special projects" are accepted. However over the subsequent six to 12 months, their observations and recommendations become less eagerly accepted and they are given the indication their work is expected per their Position/Job Description. After some time, either Management or Board may have other special projects arise but rather than use the "in-house" expertise, new external

Consultant(s) would be engaged from Consulting Firms to undertake the projects.

This is clearly Management's and the Board's prerogative and within their power to take those decisions but the dynamics are interesting to observe. After 24-36 months, the "in house" consultants are either totally transformed in to regular staff and lose their external objectivity, or leave the organization.

27   **Department Managers must learn to assume an "ownership" mentality** of their Departments and "learn and know their business", as if they were operating the business in their own capacity.

Ownership, is a legal position where real, physical, or intellectual property and assets belong to an individual or legal entity/person (shareholders, stakeholders, investors), who have the right and authority to dispose or give away basic resources of their business. But as owners of businesses, they need to know what is happening and be "tuned in" to all activities of their business. Many hospital departments (Imaging, Pharmacy, Laboratories, Rehabilitation Services, Dialysis Units, etc.), could actually function as independent business entities and be physically located outside the hospital facility. However, these services are operated within the confines of the hospital for the convenience of patients and doctors, as well as, providing income to the hospital.

So, each Department Manager/Head of Department should treat the Department as THEIR Business, as if they independently owned it, monitoring all related activities, specifically knowing the condition of all the equipment, status of supplies, inventories, and all staff working there. As "Owners", they should also know and monitor the daily/weekly/monthly workload of key pieces of equipment (e.g. CTs, MRIs, PET, lab analyzers, dialysis machines, therapy equipment, etc.), overall Department performance metrics (e.g., tests performed, prescriptions filled, therapy sessions completed, appointments scheduled and productivity levels. They should also know the operational capacity of the equipment, number and productivity of staff working, as well as status of repairs, special projects under consideration, development or implementation. Knowledge of the computer systems supporting the Department, how they work, and understanding the reports generated to determine if the information was useful. Revenue and expense information must be reviewed and monitored on a daily basis and not just month end when reports are due. Only when a Manager takes responsibility for all these components under consideration, do they know their business! Further, they should be able to meet and provide an update to Senior Management whenever they visit the Department, and be proactive in providing the information. Once they have achieved that level of "ownership" and identification with the Department's operations can they really be the Manager.

Let me share and example. During my regular "walk around" activities, I made a point to visit all the Clinical Support Departments providing services ordered by the Doctors and Specialists. We typically started out by meeting the Manager who would accompany me on my visit. During the first few visits in the Imaging Department, I would ask the Manager about the Department's workload, such as the number of MRI procedures performed in a day, a week, and month. Was workload up or down compared with the prior month, year to date, and year on year. I asked similar questions about the CT, Echo-Doppler, Fluoroscopy, the Cardiac Cath equipment. We also asked questions about their performance relative to budget, to help "pull all the activities" together. Over a period of several months the Department Manager became very well informed about the activities in the Department, and would eventually brief me on all the key workload figures for each of the pieces of equipment, and was up to date in the status of repairs, inventories, supplies, management of backlog cases (time of waiting list), budget, etc. and became comfortable enough to share with me any particular problems where they needed help, which I always made a point to follow-up for them. This created a good working relationship, and the Department Manager shared with me when I was leaving the hospital that she really appreciated the discipline that I helped to instill in her and her Department. It really works.

28   **Department Managers must recognize their "stewardship" responsibility** in operating their respective Departments.

Aligned with an Ownership mentality is the concept of Stewardship.

Stewardship, is the concept of responsibility to look after, and grow the assets (physical, financial, social, or environmental) on behalf of the Owner (shareholder, stakeholder, investors) with the expectation to preserve the principal, and improve (value add) over a period of time. As employees, this role is more onerous than Ownership, as it requires us, the employees, to take basic resources/assets and transform and optimize them on behalf of the Owners. If we fail in this aspect, we can expect to be replaced.

Senior Management (Directors, Chiefs, Division Heads, etc.), Administrators, Managers, Supervisors all share in this Stewardship role on behalf of the Owners, so they must preserve, protect, and grow assets of the organization. Therefore, all individuals in the management chain must understand the Ownership role, while exercising their Stewardship responsibilities. All individuals in the management chain must know and develop an understanding of the business, and the related metrics under their direct care with a view to optimize, or grow the business in alignment with direction of the organization, and to work together with and complement all other departments in achieving the goals and objectives of the organization.

So all Senior Staff must develop the mindset of an Owner who provides resources and assets, engages individuals to operate and manage the business and increase the value of the Owner's assets who have the right to expand, maintain, merge, or dispose of their assets.

29 When preparing a Pro-Forma, costing calculation, or determining the price of a service/product with assistance of the Finance Staff, **it is the Department, or Program Manager who owns the data**, as the Models are based on their input and understanding of what they want to achieve. **Finance is only the Facilitator.**

Oftentimes new ideas and projects, or programs are being proposed or developed with the objective for implementation, if all the internal hurdles are satisfied. Normally staff assigned to the Program Manager or a Department Head will approach the Finance Department to build a financial model to measure and reflect the incremental change or contribution to be made. The Finance staff would gather the information and assumptions from the individuals involved and use it to build the most accurate and reflective model, and observe the outcome. Based on the initial results, many iterations will follow, often requiring a revisit of the key statistic drivers and cost assumptions, and verification of data with known competitors published information. Finance may then help in generating a series of "what ifs" to give the Department a reasonable range of potential outcomes. If accepted, then it would be up to the Department to promote, and defend their recommendation to management for consideration and adoption. I always make sure Managers from the Departments are aware that the Finance staff are Facilitators, taking in the key elements and generating the outcomes, but the Departments/Project Leaders are the Owners.

So it is never acceptable for Department Heads/Managers to make a statement "the results were exclusively generated by Finance". This is important so that whatever the outcome, the Owner's takes credit for a successful outcome, or its shortfall. Finance can offer insights and suggestions for consideration to help Departments in their "model building" and may have selected relevant historical information for consideration, and final adoption, or modification by the Departments. Hopefully, at the end of the Project, after many Pro-Forma iterations, the Financial Model is realistic in terms of workload, built using the best market intelligence and cost information available, which in turns allows for a pricing structure that will satisfy the expected returns.

This approach is also relevant when there is a general review of the current detailed pricing structures, and Finance may perform certain calculations to determine what adjustments or changes to workload would be required to improve returns. Again Finance can offer observations, suggestions and options, but it is the Department that needs to re-validate the date, check market sentiment and activity, or revision of internal processes, and accept the outcomes.

30 If you are documenting the sequence of procedures performed, or developing a financial costing for services or programs, **make sure you validate the details with individuals with experience** who can confirm your approach, assumptions and thereby give you confidence on the completeness.

One of the responsibilities of a Service Department Head is to work with Finance to review the work performed and develop a "costing" of the activities performed to determine the total cost of the services being performed, and given the current or projected workload the contribution to the organization is being achieved.

In that process, the Finance Department must be engaged to prepare the required financial model to make the determination, and the Finance Department is always advised to avoid preparing the costing without detailed input from the Division or Department Manager who is knowledgeable about the internal workings and requirements. Certain procedural costings are simple and straightforward, however many product and procedure costings are complex and consume many resources, direct and indirect. Consider the following types of information required from the Department Managers or Service Providers in determining the Direct Costs:

30.1 Procedures/Products – Estimated number of products to be sold or procedures performed,

30.2 Manpower - List the Job Title and Grade of each individual involved in delivering the service or procedure, as well as the amount of "time" (in FTE or minutes) required from each participant, so appropriate cost estimates can be developed. The "time" component must include

30.2.1 preparatory work before seeing, treating, or operating on the patient,

30.2.2 actual "hands-on" time, start to finish,

30.2.3 follow-up and documentation time after the consultation, treatment, or operation,

30.2.4 as well as an allowance for "efficiency factor",

30.3 Supplies and Consumables – These are the items used in the provision of the product or service, and includes items used by the equipment (packs, scopes, special gas, cryogenics etc.), gauze, ointment, syringes, medications specific to the delivery of the service, towels, etc.,

30.4 Equipment Utilization and Operational Hours - Defining the number of hours per day, and number of days per week the equipment will be available (to determine baseline for availability and calculating workload optimization (separate costing),

30.5 Equipment Depreciation and Utilities – Identify the types of equipment required and used in provision of the services, and any costs to operate on a per procedure basis (separate costing), and allocate a portion to the procedure,

30.6 Space Requirements – Indicate the locations where the procedure(s) are to be delivered, and the "rental cost" of that space to be factored in the costing, (again separate costing).

To these Direct Costs of a product or service, Finance will add the Direct-Indirect costs (individual department administrative overhead), then make provisions for general Facility, Administrative Overheads, and required Contribution Margins. Once this is completed, the costs can be divided by the projected workload (as well as the optimum workload) to calculate a "unit cost" for the product or service which can then be used as a starting point for strategic analysis and pricing purposes.

The key point here is that all the direct numbers MUST be provided by the Department or Service provider, and Finance must validate the numbers with the Department. The Department is the "ultimate owner" of the numbers, and if the product is to be sold, or service provided, it must be based on the outcome of the costing. As part of the process, Finance should always obtain the signature of the Department staff involved in the costing process to ensure ownership.

Finally, where possible, price data should be collected from two to four other facilities offering similarly named services for comparison. However, caution must be exercised, as there may be differences in the content, due to "bundling of services" but retaining a simple procedure or service nomenclature. If your organization is the only provider of a service, your pricing should be based on the costing derived, and the organization's pricing policies, and market conditions.

31 In one's role and responsibility as a Supervisor, it is important to **maintain a degree of "professional distancing"**. Remember, it is good to work closely with your subordinates, but do not become too close or too friendly as you need to maintain a distance for purpose of "providing an objective performance assessment, promotion action, or for managing a disciplinary situation".

Professional distancing is the practice of keeping an intentional "space" between operational staff and the Supervisors, Managers, and above. A good analogy is the military structure which is designed to keep the Enlisted Men quarters and activities separate from the Officers.

Even though Supervisors, Managers and above may at times work closely with all levels of staff on projects, or even help in daily operational duties, staff must know and respect the different reporting relationships and mindful about overstepping professional boundaries. One must remember Supervisors, Managers and above will be held responsible for providing directions, as well as, accountable for outcomes achieved. Therefore, while Supervisors and Managers, and others in the hierarchy are encouraged to "go out for dinner" after a particularly difficult exercise, such as "year-end closing", successful passing of an accreditation survey, or completion of a special team project to recognize efforts, commitments and to promote "bonding" between the levels, one must avoid becoming too attached or developing emotional relationships (and the perceptions they may generate) which could impact or affect an independent, objective assessment of staff work performance. In most organizations during the annual appraisal and promotion exercises, it is the Supervisors, Managers and other Senior staff who are involved in the review process and they must be able to rank all the employees according to defined criteria and make recommendations for recognition. It is also the reason at most facilities that evaluations and recommendations need to be reviewed and supported by the "next tier up" in the Supervisory chain of command, all the way up to the CEO/MD being reviewed by their direct boss, and then their evaluation reviewed by the entire Board.

This "distancing" is also required when there is need for corrective or disciplinary action. Regardless of how well the Supervisors, Managers and others work together, if a major infraction of policy, or breech or ethics occurs, the same Supervisors, Managers, and others will be involved in administering the required disciplinary actions, ranging from verbal or written warnings, suspension, all the way up to termination, or even as far as filing a police report if the situation requires.

Similar to driving rules, remember, be professional, and maintain a safe distance.

32   Under certain conditions, it may be warranted to **put specific key staff in "golden handcuffs"** to retain their services during times of rapidly escalating compensation, to avoid disruption in an important service or Project.

During critical times, one must take special action to ensure continuity of certain projects whereby any change in key personnel could have serious negative operational and/or financial consequences. Normally we try to follow established and approved Management and Human Resource (HR) Department Guidelines on salaries and benefits. Established HR Departments will be the first to "sound the alarm" of any proposed material deviations from the approved compensation structure with various caveats that this action could impact other staff in similar positions, so this must be managed sensitively. Before taking the decision to make a special arrangement, the following criteria must be seriously considered and justified. Specifically, the total calculated cost of any increase in compensation must be less than –

32.1   Cost of the position vacancy in terms of delay in delivery timeline of the Project which could be anywhere from to six to twelve months,

32.2   Recruitment fees incurred in replacing the staff (normally one to three months of base salary in fees for most professional level staff);

32.3   Lack of new staff productivity, being oriented, educated on the corporate direction and the Project Objective, loss of momentum caused by the vacancy of the key position (could be from three to six months or more); and, "learning curve cost" time for the replacement staff to be brought "up to speed" (another six to twelve months) depending on the background of the replacement, particularly, if from a different industry than healthcare,

32.4 Further, if the job market segment is active for the particular skillset required, the organization may end up paying the same (or even higher) total compensation package in the end, while suffering all the delay, if the decision is to release the incumbent.

From the options above select the one that generates the highest number of months and multiply by the total current salary (base salary, bonuses, benefits), to determine the minimum cost of the delay. (NOTE: If the Project has high visibility and a critical implementation schedule, the number could be higher.)

However, the organization must be creative in its implementation approach. One good example where this approach was utilized, was in the IT Department during the Y2K preparation time, when a special project was in place to replace both the software and concurrently upgrade/replace the hardware to cope with the new software requirements, as well as keeping the "old" system functioning during this transition time, and while the new system was being calibrated, installed, and staff trained before the cutover. At that time, within the IT industry, demand for many staff with experience was quite high, led by the explosive growth in implementation of new software upgrades, and equipment installation to achieve a major upgrade by the year-end cutover deadline. Rather than lose the service of the IT Director/Senior Manager, and several other key staff who were intimately involved in the replacement and installation plans, we devised a modified compensation package to retain the individual(s), with a component designated as a "market adjustment" supplement (not built into the base salary component) with the caveat that as soon as the "market" caught up with the increase, the supplement would be discontinued.

This "market adjustment supplement" concept was recognized and approved. Subsequently it became a "tool" available for HR and Management and has been used in times when the market conditions created an imbalance within the prevailing salary structure for certain positions, following the certain criteria developed.

33 Organizations should make it mandatory to **develop and implement a Business Continuity Plan (BCP)** as soon as reasonably possible. This will help to protect the people, physical, and intellectual property. It is critical that the Board and Senior Management make a commitment and support the efforts required.

With the 9/11 attack in 2001 of the World Trade Center, outbreak of SARS in 2003, and a number of high profile corporate failures and scandals such as Enron, Arthur Anderson, Lehman Bros, Goldman Sachs etc., raised the recognition for being proactive and developing plans to avoid similar scandals and management failures. Aligned with that thinking, a new concept called Business Continuity Planning was emerging. The concept of Business Continuity Planning and Management was just starting to gain momentum in the US and Europe, starting in the banking industry. In 2003 developing a Business

Continuity Plan and Management with a focus on Healthcare in Singapore was the first to emerge in the ASEAN Region. The concept was to apply BCM principles to develop holistic forward thinking plans. The term "business continuity" relates to an organization having a plan(s) or framework to continue the Core Business Functions (CBF) of the organization after the company has experienced an event which could cause major disruption, or even closure of the business. The "management" component is the proactive, forward planning process, where an organization develops specific actions and responses to address a number of potential threat events which, if they occur, could deny staff access to an entire physical facility, or key departments thereby causing disruptions of key processes that prevent continuation of the core business. Initially, there was confusion when the concept of BCP for healthcare facilities was introduced. Most hospitals and healthcare facilities regularly "practiced" for situation where there were serious incidents, e.g. crashes (cars, busses, planes, and ships), building collapses, fires, etc., so there was a false sense of already "being prepared". Only once it was made clear the focus of BCP/M was to ensure the physical Hospital or Healthcare facility was ready and resilient to respond to any situation that jeopardized or threatened the continued operation of the hospital or healthcare facility structure. Denial of access to the healthcare facilities would prevent the "missions" of the various facilities to be available to treat and manage injured patients.

After the above referenced list of devastating activities from 2001 through 2003, and a new concern over potential work disruption exposure, our Board became concerned and took initiative to require the Management Team from each facility to take time and invest resources to undergo the process of developing a realistic Business Continuity Plan. The primary objective of any Business Plan is to protect and preserve the People, Property (physical facilities and assets), and Intellectual Property. In most companies having a few selected departmental "contingency plans" were considered as having a Business Continuity Plan, but that perception is wrong! Rather a Business Continuity Plan is an organization wide (holistic), location specific, integrated set of plans that can be activated in part or entirety, depending on the severity of the disruptive event! Further it needs to have necessary Policies and Procedures (or SOPs) developed and signed off by Senior Management, realistic consideration of potential outcomes, and workable strategies developed, rolled out, tested, and continuously updated by the entire facility. The P&P/SOPs must be updated whenever there is a major change in the design, internal operational structure, or workflow of the organization, which is reviewed at least once annually. It is also recommended to invest in appointing one of the "accrediting" companies that can perform an independent assessment of the organizations plan and state of readiness, and presenting a Certificate to the Board that will give them comfort that actions have been taken. However, achieving initial Certification will only be the first step, the "management" component requires constant review and testing to keep it current as new and more sophisticated threats emerge, so it is actually becomes "a long term journey".

Sadly, many small business practices, companies/organizations (GP or private medical practices, outpatient clinic groups, free standing medical services) fail to understand the principles or make plans or provisions for any disruptive event, and make the ultimate sacrifice, closing down. Actually, small and medium sized organizations can be simpler as they have fewer Departments, physical properties, and assets to protect, and could develop Business Continuity Plans/Management structure to survive a major disruptive event.

So, it is recommended that effort be expended to implement a BCP as this will help to demonstrate proper thought has been given to protect the people, plant and intellectual property of the organization, due diligence has been performed, thereby eliminating certain conditions which can "keep Board Members or Senior Management awake at night" giving "piece of mind" that the business will continue being an "ongoing concern".

34   When sourcing for equipment, **be cautious for invitations from vendors to send Member(s) of the Evaluation and Selection Work Group on a free trip** to reference site, because it can create situations that would place the Member's in a "'conflict of interest" situation.

There will be situations where certain pieces of expensive equipment will need to be acquired as a new addition to an existing facility, or a replacement for equipment past its "useful life" and encountering maintenance and support issues. In their efforts to market their products, various vendors will work with and often offer to arrange for one (or two) key individuals involved in the evaluation process of a specific Model under consideration to a reference site for the purpose of obtaining a better perspective of the features while in operation. The offer may be good from the learning perspective, but the individual(s) involved in the site visit should take various precautions to avoid any semblance of a "conflict of interest", particularly, if the vendor expresses willingness to pay for all expenses related to the site visit.

Most Boards and Senior Management have specific "ethical practices" in place to protect all parties involved, and avoid any criticism, or contentious challenges after a selection award is made. Depending on the money quantum involved in the acquisition of the equipment, any company that failed to be selected, particularly if they met the specification requirements, and may have even submitted a lower price can lodge a complaint which can delay award and installation pending resolution. It will also create negative media and reputation issues.

To avoid this type situation, as part of the replacement budget for the equipment, a provision should be made to allow for at least one to three site visits, from which any site visit expenses are to be captured and charged as a "cost of the acquisition". Should any vender be allowed to assume/pay expenses on behalf of the individuals, this can result in an expectation that the individual(s) will exert "pressure" to acquire a specific piece of equipment. So, by the organization paying for all related associated expenses, when the final selection is made, it will be based on an objective, best suited to meet the organization's need evaluation.

To address the situation and yet maintain impartiality, an offer can be made to visit a reference site by the Vendor, but the Department Head will make the determination of the Member(s) to go, and the organization will be responsible for the expenses. Upon return, a Report will be prepared and submitted to the Evaluation and Selection Work Group with their assessments and evaluation rating on their compliance, but Senior Management must take a decision whether the individuals involved can, or cannot, participate in the final "voting or selection".

Should a Department or Evaluation Team Member be sponsored (all expenses paid) by the Vendor for the reference site visit, the Member would submit a Report to the Work Group, but will be barred from "voting" when time for the Work Group to make a selection.

Following this guidance and learning on management of site visits, should there ever be any challenges relating to "conflict of interest" or improper influence issues, the organization can defend its actions and impartiality. For any further questions, advice should be sought from the organization's legal counsel.

35 Doctor's experience an **"epiphany"** upon moving into private practice. Overnight, they adopt practices and values that were previously annoying, and find they can manage their practice with the most basic of equipment, even used equipment, which was problematic while in institutional practice.

While doctors and specialists are working in public healthcare facilities, they often "want or need" specific high end pieces of equipment to perform their work, such as echo cardiographs, ultrasounds, Magnetic Resonance Imaging (MRI), and Computerized Tomography (CT) imaging equipment, as well as sophisticated lab equipment. Certain equipment pieces with multiple features and specialized software are required because of research resolution quality requirements for services being offered in institutional practice.

However, if and when the specialist decides to take up private practice, they soon realize and appreciate the cost of equipment, renovations, and often underestimate the investment required during their exit planning. As a result, they experience an "epiphany" and realize they can perform many procedures with much less sophisticated equipment than they demanded while in public/institutional practice and preserving potential investment funds for their operational expenses. There have been instances where doctors approach hospital management and offer to purchase any older pieces of equipment that the facility is planning to retire or has retired. In many instances, the retired equipment is still operational, and/or with a small investment for repairs by the Specialist, the equipment supplier can repair, upgrade, and recalibrate items in order to certify them operational and in compliance for license renewal, as the equipment can last a few more years. In fact, I had one instance where an O&G Specialist approached me (after being referred by the Purchasing Department) and requested to purchase a de-commissioned ultrasound machine. Based on the hospital's approved Disposal Policy, Net Book Value (NBV) or Trade In Value (TIV), whichever was higher was to be used as the basis to set a price. After some minor negotiation, we finally approved the sale of the ultrasound to the Specialist. Ironically, this was the same piece of equipment the specialist lobbied for replacement while maintaining his practice in the facility.

Ultimately, once their practice becomes successful, the Specialist usually upgrades their equipment; however, they will become both selective in their required features as well as price conscience of their capital investment outlay to ensure they meet their specific needs. The point of this observation is that more basic pieces of equipment can still perform without all the "bells and whistles" of newer equipment when setting up a private practice.

36 **A major difference between public and private practice**, is that in public practice, doctors strive to provide only what is really required for the medical management at the lowest cost. In private practice, doctors can provide what the patient's/parent's want, and who gladly pay.

Financial or funding methodologies influences the ways medical practice is delivered, as well as expectations of the patients seeking services.

Medical practice in the public (government, quasi government, restructured) sector often requires medical staff to rationalize medical services based on their approved annual budgets, as well as, the inventory of operational "equipment and tools" they have available to deliver services. Since public sector doctors and specialists are typically employees of a government, or government affiliated hospital, they work under various constraints with a mandate to manage and treat as many patients as possible, especially relevant during disease outbreak conditions (e.g., SARS, HFMD, multiple strains of bird flu, annual general flu, etc.), while being mindful of the related costs, so they tend to be more stringent, stretched, and practical in the use of precious resources. It is well known certain conditions are virus based versus bacteria based. Bacteria based conditions respond well with a controlled course of antibiotics and the patient condition improves quickly. Further, doctors will generally try to use an antibiotic that is both medically appropriate (not to use a super antibiotics when an earlier generation antibiotic is still effective) while also being cost effective.

However, virus based conditions are impervious to antibiotics, and most must "run their course", normally lasting five to seven days. After the doctor establishes the cause of their illness is a virus, in these instances, many public sector doctors and specialists will advise the patient or family to monitor the symptom(s) and conditions, without prescribing many tests or treatment medicines. In certain instances non-prescription medications will be recommended to help manage symptoms.

Medical practice in the private sector is driven by demand, which in the private sector, is defined as patients who are able and willing to pay for private healthcare service, as the hospitals and clinics providing private care receive little or no ongoing support from government. They are businesses, designed to deliver healthcare, and the doctors receive compensation based on the number and medical conditions of patients they manage; hospitals receive their money from providing services, equipment, and physical facilities to support the doctor's treatment requirements, as well as patient beds, nursing, and support services.

There are patients, parents, and caregivers who are not satisfied with the medical treatment or advice given at the public hospitals, and then choose to visit a private specialist or hospital to seek a "second opinion" and/or obtain further care. Since the private doctor and specialists income is derived from the patients seen and treated, to meet the expectations of their patients or families, they have the obligation to explain different treatment modalities, as well as order different tests and medications to help assuage their fears and concerns. Since the patient is willing to pay for the services rendered, the doctors will normally try to accommodate them unless the patient or their family's requests are clearly inappropriate or unethical.

Another reason certain patients, their parents, or caregivers seek services in a private hospital or clinic is to access medical services faster than what may be available in the public hospital or clinic. While every medical condition "is serious to the patient or family", medical staff in the public hospitals may classify the condition as non-urgent (versus urgent or emergency) and place the patient on a "waiting list" for an appointment, treatment, or surgery. If the patient or family perceive the wait as too long, they may want to secure services sooner, so will seek to be admitted at a private hospital to obtain the services within two to three days knowing they will be paying private rates for both the Specialist and hospital, but having their expectations satisfied and condition resolved in a much shorter time, compensates for the increased costs.

Several good examples that we have observed over the years are patients with dental problems, where root canals and other surgical interventions will be scheduled weeks in the future. Anyone who has ever experienced the pain of an impacted tooth, or other dental conditions can sympathize with a patient on the pain experienced that may need to be endured pending treatment, and appreciate why they may seek treatment in an alternative location regardless of the cost. Another example is where various joint replacement implant surgeries (shoulder, hip, knee) are "rationalized", and the patient may again be placed on a waiting list that could be months, or even years in duration before consideration, so faced with extended pain, immobility, and uncertainty they may opt for treatment in the private sector. I am sure there are many more examples.

There is no right or wrong, but there is a need to understand the reasons and drivers for patient, families, and caregivers to make decisions, and the impact of those decisions. Efforts to "blur the lines" between public and private treatment, e.g. Public-Private-Partnerships (PPPs), homecare, and new computer applications being developed, e.g. tele-medicine, and AI initiatives are being developed so as to give patients easier access to more medical treatment solutions/options at affordable rates.

37   Observation, doctors leave for private practice for three primary reasons, they are **VERY GOOD, VERY SERVICE MOTIVATED, OR THEIR CONTRACT IS NOT RENEWED........**

All Doctors and Specialists will have obtained both their basic and advanced medical skill training in either a public, private, university, or military affiliated hospital training program facility(ies). That is the normal experience gathering progression in their career development. While in public or quasi-public service, Doctors and Specialists participate in provision of services (treating patients), education (training, both in providing and receiving), and research (bench, transitional, and practical). As they mature and develop, there comes various decision points when they need to select the medical specialty where they want to spend the rest of their professional careers, and what are their personal "drivers". So, why do Doctors/Specialist leave the public, university, or military healthcare sector? There are three basic reasons.

First, there are the Specialists who are very good at what they do, and recognize they could earn a clinically satisfying and financially rewarding career by treating private patients, and who have developed an excellent reputation and built-up a referral network of Doctors while in public sector service to keep them busy. These are the "go to Specialists" in the private sector and their skills consistently generate good outcomes to justify the fees they command from their select set of patients. A certain number of these skilled Specialists would normally retain a relationship with the public or university hospitals for purposes of conducting certain research in which they have an interest, and may serve as Professors teaching selected medical courses in the University(ies).

The second group of Doctors and Specialists are those who are primarily service oriented, and interested in exclusively providing services to patients, carrying a large workload, without being fettered by teaching and research requirements. They would continue attending compulsory annual CME courses to keep current and collect the necessary points to maintain their Medical Registration and Insurance Policies current and valid. This group also provides the doctors who:

37.1 Became the private sector General and Family Medicine Practitioners, setting up their own free standing Clinics, or join an existing Group Practice,
37.2 Work as locums,

37.3 Work as in-house doctors for individual companies,
37.4 Are engaged by insurance companies to review claim payouts; or,
37.5 Are involved in pre-approval of specific medical and surgical treatments or procedures being requested,
37.6 Join or open a Consulting Firm engaged in Healthcare Consulting,
37.7 Populate medical panels and work for HMOs providing services,
37.8 Join private healthcare facilities and government entities in administrative roles and functions, etc.
37.9 Suspend their practices to raise families,
37.10 Go back to University (attend or teach),etc.

The final group are the Doctors and Specialists are those who after working in one or more of the public healthcare hospitals or facilities decides this is not their area of interest for the next "x" number of years, or the facility notes they are having difficulty in "fitting in" which causes them to reassess their direct employment arrangement in the public, and university sector healthcare environment. They have many options, such as:

37.11 Go into private practice, set up their own practice, or join an established Group practice where they can continue attending to patients in a private outpatient clinic, and obtain admitting privileges at one or more hospitals,
37.12 Work in another capacity in a healthcare facility,
37.13 Work for voluntary or charitable organizations,
37.14 Work as a locum,

37.15 Retire from direct medical delivery and work in development of software and applications; or,

37.16 Work with equipment development or marketing companies requiring either Specialists/Doctors with previous healthcare/medical service experience to ensure relevance and benefits to the equipment or marketing programs; or finally,

37.17 Go into partial (become a mentor, advisor or medical consultant) or complete retirement.

Most doctors in public or university healthcare system are given "three to six year employment contracts" after which their performance and contributions will be reviewed by a panel, and their contract will either be renewed, or they may decide they want to leave for whatever reason to pursue other interests, so they will be released. This approach allows Doctors and Specialists an opportunity to exit public/university/military systems (without losing face) while helping provide, replenish and build up the private sector pool of Doctors and Specialists. Their exit will create openings for "a new wave of next generation" medical staff entering the system, and/or allow internal promotions in the public sector since many public sector positions (FTEs) are normally limited by their budgets. Non Specialist Doctors can leave after completion of their medical training to enter the private General Practitioner (GP)/Family Practitioner (FP) sector, while Specialists normally exit the public system between the ages of 35-45 years to allow sufficient time to build up their practices. Surgeons in the past have had to be concerned over their ability to perform operations, meeting the demands of being constantly "on call" and usually made plans to reduce their workload or take on partners when they reach the ages of 55-60 years; however nowadays with the introduction of "robotic" and AI devices to assist or perform detailed and delicate surgery, the surgeons may be able to continue performing surgeries for a longer period of time.

For the Consultant Grade Specialists, and Senior Grade Consultant Specialists (or their equivalent titles in different countries) who remain with public sector hospitals and facilities, they can be exposed to a mix of duties, obtain access to a wide variety of medical conditions they can study and treat, enjoy benefits such as, "covered" conference, annual, sick, holiday leave time, as well as, individual/family medical, personal life/accident, disability, and in some instances, med-mal insurance coverage. They also can perform specialized procedures and have opportunities to access some of the latest technological equipment, using "cutting edge" methodologies, or introducing transitional/translational research applications, conduct pure research, and yet have sufficient time to write and present papers in areas of their particular interest. A few of these Specialists can actually be the best and internationally renowned in their respective field often working with, and supporting private sector Specialists who have extremely complex cases, or collaborate in research and teaching as Professors in Universities.

38   A doctor with **great technical skills**, but lacking in the personal touch, or bedside manner, will fail or have difficulty with the patients; however a doctor with **good technical skills** but great bedside manners will succeed building a good practice; but the doctor who has **both great technical skills and demonstrates great bedside manners** will gain

respect and recognition from his patients, peers, and community!

Over the years, I have observed, listened, and identified Specialists with various combinations of technical skills and Emotional Quotient (EQ). EQ relates to the Specialists interactive, and interpersonal communications, i.e. talking with the patient and/or relatives, taking time to explain all the procedures, expected outcomes (both good and bad), so the patient has the necessary information and can make informed decisions on what they want to do, and after all the treatments and procedures are completed the Specialist/Doctor takes interest in the patient's follow-up care until they are completely discharged

There are some Specialists/Doctors with great technical skills but lack or are on the low end of the EQ scale, and have an attitude of "take it or leave it" with regards to their approach or methodology, which results in denying patients who need help with the best medical care. Some of these Specialists are ones who I would personally go to (or have my family members) if I had a serious problem and wanted the best chance of proper treatment or survival. However, as I am aware of their lack of EQ we can tolerate their blunt and sometimes caustic remarks and approach in order to secure their services. Unfortunately, there are many potential patients who cannot tolerate this treatment attitude approach, and the Specialist will have a good, albeit limited practice. This Specialist tends to thrive best in an institutional setting, as they have many other support staff, especially nurses, who can compensate for their shortcomings, by offering explanations and can manage the referrals they will receive.

There is another group of doctors with good technical skills, and even better EQ skills and they tend to attract many patients into their practices. While their technical skills are good, they may not be on par with the Specialist with great technical skill but poor EQ; however, for many conditions which are straight forward enough the good technical skills are sufficient to treat the patient, and the patients feels they have had a great experience with the Specialist, and will refer other individuals who could become potential patients.

Finally, you have the special group of Specialists who have great technical skills and have developed a great set of EQ skills - the best of both attributes. For this type Specialist, the patients will queue up to be seen and treated by them, regardless of how long they have to wait for their appointment, not grumble over any long waits, and gladly settle their accounts with no questions asked.

39   It is wrong to conclude that any doctor or nurse who demonstrates and excels in medical, and patient management skills, will make an equally excellent administrator, to be moved up the organizational hierarchy; **in many instances their best work is in direct patient care and treatment.**

There is a general misunderstanding that a clinician or nurse who has worked over the years to develop their clinical and nursing skillsets and have an excellent reputation and medical outcomes with patients will also make the individual an excellent clinical or nurse administrator, or even more challenging an equally excellent hospital level Administrator. Many doctors and nurse who excel in patient care and treatment become well known because they have a passion for their profession, so they perform their best work in their chosen specialty or service. They may rise to the top of their field, and even "cover" as a Department Head or higher for a short time; however, their best work is still with patients, and if they are promoted from the direct care environment to assume administrative responsibilities on a permanent basis, may become disenchanted and fail to perform as expected. Administration and medical careers are both professions, and succeeding in medical management does not automatically translate to being able to succeed as an Administrator, when all they want to do is provide service to patients. There are Specialists and nurses who after years of clinical service become interested in administration and believe they can "add value" in a hospital or healthcare entity by moving up in the healthcare environment and providing direction, and management because they understand the environment and system. In those instances the doctors and nurses can "relate" to both the medical/surgical and nursing staff, understanding their problems and potentially come up with solutions for the betterment of the Specialists and nurses, and that is a good outcome for everyone. But for the clinicians and nurses who really enjoy treating patients, we must respect their wishes, and management must provide meaningful career paths so they will continue to be motivated, and the patients benefit.

40   The best way to **get doctors** to "buy into" an idea or project is to get them **to think the idea was theirs**.

Over the years as an Administrator in various healthcare related roles, we Administrators often have good ideas or concepts to improve clinical process to help medical staff; however, many ideas were presented but often most were dismissed by the medical staff, particularly when in groups, with the statements that it cannot be done and "Administrators do not understand clinical aspects or it's a waste of their time", so the ideas fail to be recognized, and subsequently deferred. To overcome the dismissive approach it was necessary to work with a few Specialists/Doctors who are willing to take time and effort to listen and learn about the suggestions, discussing their strengths and weaknesses, and if they ultimately make sense let the Specialist/Doctor raise the ideas for discussion amongst their medical peers in an appropriate forum and in most instances the ideas will be accepted, based on the "source" of the idea. Once the Specialist/Doctors perceive the changes were brought about by their peers, the same Administrators are engaged to help facilitate implementation, which was the objective in the first place. Once adopted, the concepts can easily be shared and spread amongst different hospitals in the general area. A good example was the introduction of the Clinical Pathways. Various presentations were made to medical staff, who took the position this would lead to "cookbook medicine" and medical staff needed independence to apply their skills without Clinical Pathways. Over time several Specialists were introduced to the concepts, understood the benefits, and studied the documented improvements (evidence based medicine) in outcomes, the concept was introduced again by Clinicians who became the promoters and it was ultimately adopted, and has proven to work.

41 Senior Medical staff and Administrators of Hospitals with proper OR/OTs and support services **should**

make efforts to enter an Agreement/Arrangement to offer "back-up" services to General Practitioners and Specialists operating individual private practices or in structured Outpatient or Ambulatory Care facilities in the community.

There will always be situations at a GP or Specialist Clinic in the community, where patients present or develop a condition that requires more equipment, skillsets, staffing, supplies, etc., than their community based facilities can provide. The medical conditions may be the result of a complication arising from a routine GP or Specialist Out-patient or Ambulatory Day Care procedure, or due to a patient/family seeking medical help because of an accident e.g. severe trauma (limb, head injury), fever, infection or other condition. In interest of the patient, the individual doctor practices, as well as, the Outpatient and Ambulatory Care facilities, Hospital Management and stand-alone service providers should actively enter into Agreements to provide an integrated "network of medical service providers" whereby patients can be readily transferred to the most appropriate environment for treatment, which is usually a Hospital setting.

Advance planning and knowing the medical services provided by the respective Hospital(s) in the local community, or region, and promoting an Agreement/Arrangement allows both the Hospital and Doctors to have a strategy and "back door" to initiate continued treatment. A Hospital's 24 Hr. Clinic or A&E/ER can be alerted while the patient is in the process of being transferred and other services can be put on stand-by, i.e. imaging, lab, bed, OR/OT if necessary. When managed correctly, the patient is given the best chance for survival. This approach has the added benefit of aligning GPs, Specialists with the Hospitals and developing and strengthening a strong referral network amongst all parties.

42. Senior Clinical, Chairman of Medical Board or equivalent, and Senior Hospital Management, CEO, or equivalent must always **be sensitive to "clinical' politics**, and take measure to moderate.

Hospitals and healthcare facilities are comprised of a "critical core" of Specialists who have come together in order to provide quality services to patients. It is their intention to provide a "network" of Specialists so Members can provide ready referrals within the Hospital or Healthcare facility, and bolster both their internal workloads, as well as support the organization. This supportive relationship is considered a positive political environment, building a strong working relationship and promoting Team building.

However, there are instances where differences arise between two or more Specialists and/or Administration over specific practices, issues, rules, or management policies.

For personal disagreements (within work or outside) between Specialists, to show their dissatisfaction, Specialists are known to refer patients to external Specialists, when the expertise of another Specialist is required, yet there is a Specialist within the Hospital or healthcare facility who may be equally or more qualified; but due to their personal relationship differences, may "cloud their clinical judgement" on who is the best for managing the patient's condition.

A disagreement can also occur between the Specialist(s) and Administration if certain processes or policies are in question. An example would be Specialist(s) who schedules appointments for their patients at another Hospital or external service for an MRI, CT, Angiography, etc. when one is provided within the Hospital's Imaging Department but the Specialist perceives need for a more powerful one, when a basic or mid-level one is provided by the Hospital and is all that is required. This external scheduling results in inconvenience to the patient, loss of revenue within the Hospital, and a dangerous breakdown in the internal referral system. If unchecked, these practices affect morale of the Hospital's Specialists, and their performance which in turn leads to separate networks being built.

Therefore, Chairman of the Medical Board, and perhaps the hospital's CEO, need to call for an emergency Medical Staff Meeting (or add to the Agenda of an upcoming Medical Board Meeting) to learn about and discuss the reasons for the emerging practices, and take efforts to resolve the issue/feud, and recommit the Specialists support their fellow Team Members and the organization that is providing Specialists the necessary tools and environment to function. Alternatively, if just emerging or limited between a few Specialists, or a few Specialists and Administration, a "one-on-one" discussion may be more appropriate approach.

The purpose of highlighting this Observation is to create awareness on actions to initiate if a situation is brought to your attention, and encourage Senior Management to be proactive in efforts to resolve these problems before permanent damage occurs. With a large number of professional Medical staff affiliated with the Hospital or Healthcare facility, over time it is inevitable that issues will arise. So, the faster they are identified and addressed, the better!

> 43 Remember the **3Rs** of Financial Reviews, Activities, and Decisions -
>
> 43.1 **RELATIONSHIPS** - Everything is related, in cause and effect, proportion/percentages. Look and compare the changes, before and after an assumption or parameter is changed
>
> 43.2 **REASONABLENESS** - Every outcome should approach/approximate and tend toward an expected outcome, as well as making sense. Investigate anything that appears outside that scope; and,
>
> 43.3 **RATIONALE** - Every change and effect should be logically defensible

Every decision taken within an organization has a financial impact. The impact may be to increase revenues, reduce expenses, achieve a "zero sum" adjustment, or a combination thereof, so, there is always a cause and effect situation. That is why financial and accounting staff ask questions in order to perform analysis to determine the "incremental" impact of any decision. That is also why Managers and Senior Staff need to be sensitive to any changes in prices, costs, workload performed, legislative/regulatory actions, and Ministry/Department of Health Policies and Guidelines.

All actions taken are **related**. A great example of this statement can be observed from a technique learned over the years, called "intensity factor" which basically demonstrates any changes to key "workload drivers" will have a "ripple effect" throughout the organization, and across departments. This allows for design of budget and Pro-Forma document Worksheets which allow for assumptions to be made and then update the financial model. For example, if admission activities change, either up or down, it is most likely due to cumulative effect in the number of outpatients treated (in Clinics, 24 Hour Accident & Emergency/Emergency Department services, or a shift in Ambulatory Day Treatment/Surgery workload), which will result in incremental relational changes in the workload from all Departments providing services to support each admitted patient. Every admission, will impact on demand for beds (inpatient or observation), Prescriptions (medications/drugs), Diagnostic/Therapeutic imaging services (X-rays, MRI, CTs, fluoroscopy, etc.), Lab Tests (extensive array of services), Operating Room/Theatre space, Therapy treatments (physio, occupational, speech, respiratory, psychological), as well as, meals, and a host of other direct services supporting each admission (laundry/linen, environmental/housekeeping, patient transport, etc.). In the aggregate, the impact of any sizable increase or decrease will resonate throughout organization because they are all inter-related, and they will be impacted, requiring more or less in staffing, supplies, consumables, materials and equipment.

The point is that when making strategic budgetary changes whether in prices, or workload, one should be mindful of, and ensure all areas providing support flex and adjust according to new levels (plus or minus) of service required. This is most critical during the annual budgetary process when major new programs are taken into consideration, as operational or strategic changes are factored into projections. Minor changes during the year can normally be accommodated, but in subsequent years must be analyzed and taken into consideration. Any new positive revenue generating processes and programs are normally approved after stringent review and evaluation any time during the fiscal year.

Along with the relationships comes **reasonableness**. There is the need to ensure the expected results are reasonable. This is the process of ensuring all the projected changes "filter" through to the different departments producing results are consistent with the expected outcome. This is important as the numbers developed in isolation for new programs, or other changes may not be integrated, but once the changes are "plugged in" results may occur that create outcomes that appear to be "out of alignment". This type situation frequently occurs when certain "hard coded" instructions are imbedded in a software program, and fail to flex with the changes being made, resulting in numbers and do not make sense in terms of expectation. Hence, it is always good practice to manually calculate a "ballpark figure" of the expected incremental impact and match the resultant figures to determine if the system is aligned and working correctly. If the results fail this "reasonableness review", the first thing to do is to have the IT staff look into the software code, line by line. Therefore, one should validate the expectations by reviewing the before and after results to determine if they are "in alignment" to the expected outcome of the proposed/planned changes. If there is still a material outcome difference, it may require a complete review of the assumptions, and the relationships with the necessary rework.

Finally, everything done should be logically defensible and have proper **rationale**. Does the change being proposed make sense for the Organization, the Department(s) while supporting the overall strategic objectives set by the Board. Understand the reasons for making the changes and ensure they align with corporate or facility objectives, and that they contribute to the overall performance of the organization in a positive manner. At times certain decisions may take longer than one year to implement and yield the benefit because necessary actions leading up to the implementation must be addressed in sequence, e.g. construction of a new building/wing, renovation of an outpatient clinic, development of a new service requiring specialty trained staff and protocols, acquisition of special equipment, and/or obtaining approvals/inspections from various regulatory entities. But looking forward in the workload and financial projections, there should be clear indication the decisions taken were correct. Key Management and Department Head staff must be committed and take ownership of the actions to be taken. Finally, with regards to rationale, efforts should be made to validate the proposals. For proposal with external impact, e.g. prices for services, efforts should be made to obtain prices for similar services from other hospitals or facilities. Compare the results with proposed changes to determine if they are defensible from a market perspective. If this is a completely new service, without comparison, then decisions can be taken for introduction given the "first mover" principles and market leader focus. With infrastructure or operational procedure changes which are strictly internal, then estimates of current costs to provide the service or product should be compared with the savings or reallocation of resources to analyze the "cost vs benefits" of making the change, and proceed accordingly.

While this explanation appears long, with use of templates, discussion, "homework" performed by the key owners, and with decent market intelligence, it is very manageable and ultimately should become part of the organization's culture.

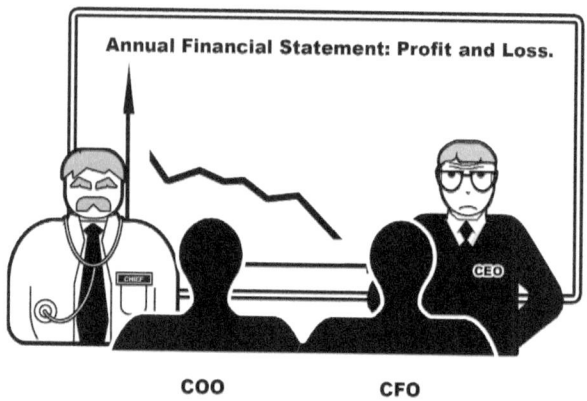

 I believed you misunderstood me!
I wanted us to achieve "Non-Profit Status", and not to be "Non Profit"!

44   One must understand that being **an organization with a "Non Profit" status**, is a tax concession granted by the recognized government Tax Assessment Authority. It is to waive tax on earnings/surpluses generated by provision of core services in the approved industry, e.g. public healthcare provision activities, and allows for any surpluses to be retained and used for expansion/provision of similar services. It **does not mean that the business/organization can or should be operated at a loss**, as being non-financially viable will ultimately cause the organization to fail without other sources of income.

Periodically we must educate staff who equate the concept of an organization having "non-profit" status as being a facility that can operate at a loss (i.e., total revenues/funding sources are less than total expenses). Short term situations of operating at a loss can occur, such as in new "start-ups/acquisitions" or due to an economic downturn, are sustainable for a limited period of time; however, this should never translate into a long term, steady state expectation of the hospital, as they would go out of business. The concept of "non-profit" status is a government income tax authority classification in most countries whereby the earnings generated from the provision of medical services to patients are exempt from normal income tax exposure. For clarity, the net income (revenue less expenses) from non- hospital or affiliated healthcare related services/products not provided or generated by the hospital is subject to income tax, such as, rental income from any commercial space leased out in the facility, sales of any products in a hospital operated general retail services (e.g. commercial pharmacy, rehab supplies, and equipment, food courts/cafeterias, auditorium fees collected for externally sponsored activities, etc.), parking fees collected, management or professional consulting services fees charged to external organizations, or other services not involving direct patient care within the hospital. The purpose of the "non-profit" status is to allow the eligible hospitals/healthcare facilities to build up their financial reserves by retaining any positive earnings/surpluses and having them available to reinvest those amounts into planned equipment replacement or upgrading, improving or expanding patient care programs; thereby, reducing the amount of funds the facilities would need to borrow for equipment and/ or expansion with the expectation to lower financial interest payments which becomes an operating cost passed along to the patient. This exemption is normally extended to government or community affiliated healthcare facilities, religious, recognized charitable or welfare organizations. It is not normally applicable to privately owned and operated hospitals and related businesses. Governments may offer alternative tax treatment or incentive schemes to encourage healthcare related investments in the private sector.

So just recognize, having a "non-profit" status is a tax related situation, and not an operational condition.

45 Remember, from a financial perspective, **any organization/department can "live within its defined, approved budget"** as required by its Board and internal management guidelines. It will only be an issue of the quantity, quality, and scope of services/products to be provided. All or parts of these elements will be modified, consolidated, or sacrificed in the process. In these instances, **Management must identify and focus on preserving its organization's Critical Business Functions (CBF)**, and act accordingly.

A budget is a plan, based on strategic objectives, management alignment, and service/performance expectations. An organization level budget can be prepared and approved by the Board at designated Directors/Trustee Meetings with all the assumptions, goals, objectives, and proposed financial structure to achieve the desired outcomes. During the course of the year, material, new assumptions and/or programs may be implemented and the impact should to be taken into consideration, so management may call for another "working" budget to be produced, reflecting the latest directions for consideration and adoption if all the necessary hurdles are satisfied. These reviews are typically prepared on a quarterly or six month basis.

Conversely, in times where the economy is slowing down, market conditions change, service demand reduces, funding from various grants or other external support is scaled down, it will become necessary to re-examine, and recast the budget based on the updated information. As a financial model, the budget can be modified to provide structure and a roadmap for the balance of the year, and in preparation for development of the subsequent year's budget. It is all a matter of adjusting the workload, performance and expectations; however, in that process, attention and care must be given to preserving and prioritizing the Critical Business Functions (CBF) of the organization ensuring the necessary service and treatment standards are achieved for the revised number of patients to be managed. Workload in all departments in the organization should then be adjusted, up or down, in response the new or revised targets and available funding.

As indicated earlier, any budget can be modified by making selected changes in four key assumption variables:

45.1 Quantity/Workload (numbers of patients to be seen or treated),

45.2 Quality (duration and extent of treatment services to be provided),

45.3 Service Expectations (standards, time related issues, and amenities provided), and, finally,

45.4 Financial Resources (money available from whatever sources). While in many instances it is easier to adapt to positive improvements and growth situations, but the "mettle" of the organization's staff is tested during times of reduction in services i.e. economic cycle downturns, or political policy type decisions that affect the organization which need to be taken into consideration, and revising the budget accordingly.

There are many methodologies and strategies that can be implemented to achieve the desired results, and staff must be briefed and instructed on ways to answer the actions taken.

46 Companies need to adopt a policy of "**pricing services and products according to the market where the services and products are being provided and sold**", and not the market where the services or products were developed.

At various times, I have noticed prices for equipment, medications/drugs, hardware and software that are ordered and purchased from reputable companies based on the pricing structure in the country of origin/manufacture, and applying the relevant currency exchange rate to the product. At times, this results in instances where items or services become too expensive for the medical facility, particularly in developing countries, to acquire or introduce. If the company wants to enter a new market, the company must be willing to make certain pricing concessions to gain entry into a particular market. One can learn from great marketing and fast food service industry leaders, who modify their prices to be more reflective of local pricing and cultural sensitivities, particularly when companies are trying to enter a new market. This approach should be raised to the companies who may tender their products and services for serious consideration. While they may not be able to reduce to completely match the local pricing structure level, they may be able to reduce the pricing sufficiently to attract several potential customers to seriously consider the products if the quality and reputation of the provider warrants. From the provider perspective, discounts offered can be taken as marketing expenses, and the company can target one or two Healthcare facilities to become "Reference/Referral Centers/Sites" to showcase their range of products to other interested potential customers in the region, who can visit and learn about the products, observe them, understand the benefits and features, and then take decisions on whether to acquire the new product or services and negotiate a "package". Otherwise the company trying to enter the market and establish a foothold will be by-passed and their product will neither be visible nor available in their target market, even if they are very good. Over time, after establishing a customer base changes can be made to adjust pricing.

Another important related component for consideration is that when a company takes a decision to expand into new markets, they must be committed to stay there and make a presence for a number of years. Too many companies try to expand during good economic times without that long term view, and when economic times go through their inevitable cycles, many companies will want to "pack up and leave" with a view and promise to return when the economic market conditions improve. This philosophy is flawed, and the company will lose credibility with customers, as most potential customers want to work with companies who are prepared to be present for the long term. Just consider what happens if products are sold, services delivered, but the long term support is no longer present. What message does that send to current or potential customers? What happens to the ongoing warranty, and support services? What happens to the business lost due to lack of support? Visibility and ongoing support plays an important role in both product and service selection, and after sales support. Make sure all these aspects are discussed, then plan and negotiate accordingly.

Consolidating and having Regional Headquarters to service a number of countries, may work for larger items, but all companies should plan to have "in-country" representation, either direct or via an "appointed agent" scheme at an in-county registered office or company where knowledgeable staff can be contacted, meet with customers in a timely manner, respond and resolve any product/service support issues for products and services already delivered. Further, keep in mind the location where any disputes are to be adjudicated, so legal/court disputes in a "far away" location, versus in the country where products and services were provided, also matters.

Two key points supporting this Observation - price your Products and Services based on the physical country location where products or services are delivered; and, ensure one has a long term view in maintaining an active presence in the country as long as one has sold any products or services that may need to be maintained.

47   Be sensitive when increasing medical staff in any clinical specialty to meet growth and budget

projections. Every new Specialist added will potentially dilute workload from existing staff, so increases must be tactful and with understanding and support from the current clinicians.

After opening or assuming operation of a hospital/healthcare Facility, there should be a Board approved strategy for recruitment of additional "admitting" Clinical Specialists (medical and/or surgical) to the hospital or healthcare facility. The decision activation points are normally determined by defined clinical "workload trigger points". When opening a new facility, or introducing a new medical specialty or service to an existing facility, clinical management must have a plan on the size and type of the services to be provided and introduced, the number of internal FTEs to be engaged or independent Specialists to be given admitting rights, allowing clinicians sufficient "protected time to grow practices", through careful monitoring of workloads. It is good practice for the initial Specialists of a particular discipline joining the facility, to be briefed on the Clinical Department's workload plans and expectations, with timetables to grow the Specialist's workload, and agree on the workload trigger points when another Specialist is to be recruited. This should be made clear in terms of the Department size to be developed, clinic space to be provided, as well as giving existing Specialists sufficient time to grow their individual practices. Metrics, such as number of patients being treated daily, waiting list (days, weeks, months) for initial and follow-up appointments, admissions, as well as actual overall workload targets need to be taken into consideration, otherwise there will be an unhealthy conflict (professional competition) created amongst the Specialists which could impact the morale and referral network/patterns within and around the hospital or healthcare facilities. Be sensitive to the number (FTEs), fulltime/part-time Specialists being recruited to join and complement existing Specialist Departments/Services, support staff required to achieve workload target for new budget approved programs. If Specialists are independent, the number of other Specialists of the same discipline, offering the same sub-specialty services can result in reduction of their individual workloads, and dilute their income potential, so this may become an issue unless they only plan to "work part-time", based on constraints of where they are currently working.

Growing a program and adding Specialists is a "good problem" to have, however it must be managed in a planned, professional manner, and sensitive to the current staff or affiliates.

48 Beware of **land offers in exchange for majority ownership** of a healthcare facility.

Over the years, as an individual in Senior Management roles, especially CEO, and COO, I have been approached by various businessmen who want to build a hospital or healthcare facility. When asked what they want to achieve, what would be their contribution, the answers received were they "want to be part of providing the people a hospital for a variety of reasons"; and, their contribution would be a plot of land on which to build the facility, for which in return they would be given 50-60% equity ownership of the entire facility; and, whoever they "partner" with would be responsible for providing all facility construction, and equipment funding, as well as working capital for operations of the facility for a specified number of years.

This type proposal must be analyzed based in context of the actual location and plot size and building ratio of the proposed land to be provided to satisfy the 50-60% equity ownership expectation. If the proposed land site was in prime development area of the city with sufficient residential population size, density, and personal income profile to support their needs at a private hospital, then it would capture our attention. It would also need to have as many as possible of community infrastructure requirements implemented or "under development" for the proposed site location and should include communication (telephone, internet), power (one or more feeds from different power grids), sewerage system, and waste water treatment systems, waste (general and biohazardous) collection, and removal using proper disposal (landfill, burial, incineration), adequate drainage system, development of access roads (both primary and secondary), public transport (bus, mass transit system, airport, taxi, ferry/boat terminals) for ease of access, and necessary government infrastructure for immigration clearances (if applicable) as well as proper, approved zoning. Only when all these components are addressed and answers obtained, can proposed equity figures in that range be considered as an opening point for negotiation.

However, based on both my and other professionals experience, in most instances where this proposed land provision, equity ownership arrangement has been raised was in under developed, and developing countries for a plot of land in an undeveloped or undeveloped piece/tract of land located some distance from a "major" city development and often isolated. The perception being that the hospital or healthcare facility will be part of a "magnet of key services" to attract and facilitate development of a residential community to migrate into a particular direction.

This assessment may be accurate from a long term perspective, perhaps in eight or more years in the future, but would not be suitable for a current investment situation. Further, as part of due diligence, it is important to look for solid evidence of progress towards installation of the necessary community infrastructure, as indicated above, to be in some phase of active development to even make this type arrangement worth consideration in the future.

The other major problem with the proposal, besides being rather financially "unbalanced", is that it would be operationally difficult to attract manpower, i.e. doctors, specialists, and other healthcare professionals (nurses, therapists, clinical support professionals, administrators, etc.) to work in such an isolated environment without a good physical and corporate referral infrastructure to make the hospital project succeed, so basically the Project may have the Developer's good intentions at heart, however the timing is not conducive for the Project's success. The first thing the Developer should do is invest in engagement of a Consulting Firm (Healthcare and/or Financial, eg., KPMG, Deloitte, PWC, etc.) to perform a comprehensive Feasibility Study to identify the hurdles that will need to be overcome, and perhaps a realistic estimate of timing. This will allow for development of a Financial Pro-Forma Model to test the assumptions. If the Developer still decides to proceed with the Project without following this recommendation, they will be at risk of "wasting their money", and with a high probability of failure.

So, for all the reasons and concerns shared above, one should be very wary of land offers in exchange for majority ownership of a healthcare facility.

49 Medical staff in both outpatient and inpatient setting should view patients as valuable resources and provide quality medical care over the patient's lifetime journey and make efforts to ensure the continuum of care is appropriate as this will ensure a steady stream of financial contributions to the healthcare Provider. **Never look at attendances/appointments as "one off" contacts or consultations with a patient, but take a "holistic" long term perspective.**

Regardless of whether you are serving public or private patients, as a GP or Specialist, besides the patient's expectation for delivery of quality clinical care, and communication, medical staff and other professionals serving patients should treat the patients as "long term", recurring recipients of care. One should work toward building a relationship where patients/customers will seek specific Doctor/Specialists services because of a good meaningful encounters, treatments, and outcomes. Further the patient/customer is also a powerful source of referrals and important to both the individual Doctor/Specialist in building up their practices, but also the hospital's or clinic's business as it attempts to provide a comprehensive range of basic and advanced support services to address the Doctors and Specialists needs who have committed themselves to the organization and have been granted admitting/treatment privileges.

With the correct attitude, this approach will be "win-win" situation for both, but to make it so, requires awareness to treat each patient with respect, dignity, and attention so the patient/customer appreciates and perceives the sincerity and completeness in delivery of care. A simple example to illustrate this concept is the Obstetric-Gynecological (Obs/Gyne)

Specialist. In most instances a female will be seen and treated by the Obs/Gyne Specialist for any gynecological related issues during her teen/young adult, and adult years, up to the point of pregnancy, then Obstetric related services are provided by the Specialist. Subsequent to delivery, the female will be back to receiving Gyne related services between and after pregnancies, for the rest of her life. If the Specialist takes proper care of his/her patient, she will be a lifetime "customer". Looking objectively, this one patient could generate one to two clinic visits per year, over a conservative period of 40-50 years, and could be managed for one to three pregnancies and deliveries over the same period. So, it is easy to visualize this relationship lasting for many years. Further, it can even generate referrals for additional patients to the Specialist. Multiply this by as many patients the Specialist can realistically support in their practice to arrive at the "big picture" opportunity. This will be to the individual patient's benefit, as well as, the long term interest of Specialist to retain the patient over their life.

While other medical specialties may have shorter interactive treatment periods, looking after the patients for their primary medical conditions, and building a rapport will result in continued preference selection for treatment, and confidence in information shared and referrals made by the Doctors and Specialists. Every medical practitioner should review their respective practices in this manner.

50 Whenever people complain about the increasing cost of healthcare, it is important that we educate them that **manpower cost constitutes from 40-65% or more of a healthcare facility's operating costs.**

Staff are professionals who have invested many years to achieve their skills to be able to treat patients in a professional manner after a proper diagnosis.

Healthcare is a service industry, largely dependent on manpower for the diagnosis and treatment of patients. Specifically, most hospitals and healthcare providers in developed countries expend between 40% and 65% of their total operating budget in manpower related costs (salaries, and benefits), in hospitals that are professionally managed, following recognized, proven treatment standards, protocols, with acceptable workloads, and staffing ratios. In emerging and less developed countries, this ratio may differ, usually due to shortfall of professional staff, high costs of importing equipment, medical supplies, consumables, and pharmaceuticals, as well as different philosophies in patient management. Technology may also contribute to the cost via depreciation and amortization of expensive high tech equipment, and computer systems (hardware and software). Variable operating costs need to be managed and balanced to provide the best medical outcomes, while minimizing risk of unplanned patient visits/re-admissions for continued treatment, while fixed costs relating to building depreciation, maintenance, interest, insurance, and utilities contribute to the balance of expenses.

Patients and families naturally want the best care for themselves or their loved ones, so there is a cost to attract, and retain reputable and qualified individuals. Most healthcare costs, and prices/fees are indexed to the local Consumer Price Indexes (CPI) for inflation plus some consideration for technology improvement. So, it is important to educate users on the composition of healthcare costs. In the private sector there is another cost to be considered, the element of shareholder returns for their investment in the business. This must be given proper consideration since the shareholders made an investment, which provided money for many services, and allows patients greater access to healthcare facilities and services, so even their efforts and foresight must be rewarded. Without the private sector to offer options to the community, the entire burden of healthcare provision for all the population would become the sole burden of the government.

Government owned and operated facilities face the same constraints and expenses as the private sector, so if government had to provide 100% of the healthcare services it would dilute precious resources, and lead to rationing of services. So, there is an important role for reputable private hospital and healthcare facilities to complement government services, and work together.

51 Be aware of the concept "Duty of Care" which is a legal and moral principle of responsibility that holds medical professionals accountable in provision of healthcare services. The **more senior the medical professional by education, training, experience, and title, the greater the obligation they have to anticipate and manage potential outcomes,** by performing tests and procedures which result in a diagnosis which allows selection of an appropriate treatment plan(s) for the patient's condition. As a result, medical bills (outpatient and inpatient) for services of the Specialists meeting those qualifications and expectation will increase accordingly, over the

doctors providing care at the primary level (GP, Polyclinic, or their equivalent).

Many families and patients for various reasons believe it is best to go to the most experienced (top) group of doctors for their very first appointment, rather than enter the healthcare system at the lower(est) level even if the underlying condition has yet to be identified. Further they then provide negative feedback and comment on long wait times, and high, or rising cost of treatment and care in the healthcare industry when they are contributing to the condition by their decision to bypass the established structure.

In most countries, there is a defined, primary, secondary, and tertiary/quaternary care hierarchical structure, and looks like a pyramid, with more doctors and staff at the lower levels whose training and roles are to address less severe conditions, and common problems and help determine if a condition should be reviewed by one or more Specialists, preferable at a secondary level hospital or healthcare facility, reserving referrals to tertiary/quaternary care facilities for the most complex of cases. This is both a responsible approach of using limited and precious healthcare services, and ensuring cost effectiveness.

Treatment by a primary care physician/doctor only requires the doctor to test and treat for the obvious condition. Their tests ordered and treatments provided will reflect their diagnosis. Should their treatment be ineffective, additional tests can be ordered to explore other options. If they are not able to resolve the issue, then they will issue a referral letter (or make a call and arrange an appointment) to a Specialist from either a secondary or tertiary tier facility for continued follow-up as that facility will have doctors with specialty training (Specialists), who focus on exotic, and esoteric conditions, and have access to more sophisticated equipment (laboratories, imaging), and medications. The primary care physician, or the secondary tier Specialist can provide a summary of a work-up already performed along with relevant test results, as well as observations, to complement the more in-depth testing and procedures to be ordered.

Given the concept of "duty of care", the more specialized the doctor is in their respective fields, the greater the obligation the Specialist will have to "rule out" any other potential cause(s) of the symptoms being experienced by the patient, so they will order more tests, and procedures to formulate a "working" diagnosis, and appropriate treatment. So using an extreme case of a patient suffering from a cold or flu, if they went to the primary physician, the bill will be substantially lower, than if the individual went directly to a Specialist, who would then be obligated to conduct more tests, and procedures to eliminate other potential causes having similar symptoms. The implication (both professional and legal) of the Specialist's failure to identify and isolate any other potential cause(s) for consideration in their diagnosis and treatment plan is substantial. Consequently, the patient/family will face a bill that is substantially larger.

The message to share and promote is to use the healthcare hierarchy of care from primary to tertiary care in a proper manner, to reduce waiting time, costs, and to ensure all doctors, from primary care Physicians to Specialists are used in the most effective manner. They are a precious resource to the community.

While doctors were selected for this explanation, the same principle of "duty of care" applies to all clinical staff within the organization (e.g. nurses, therapists), in all support service departments (environmental, maintenance, food, etc.) of the hospital or healthcare facility, including administration and outsourced services etc., with increasing individual obligations based on their ascending positions.

52. **Specialist Referral networks require years of development, and are sensitive to a number of factors** which must be taken into consideration when recruiting Doctors and Specialists for a new facility, e.g., hospital, medical clinic grouping. Even simple physical location changes of an office can have material impact on their business and makes it as challenging as if just opening a new practice.

It is naïve for any Hospital Developer or new hospital Owner/Operator to expect by virtue of building a new facility, it will automatically attract Doctors and Specialists who will "fill up the hospital" with patients in a relatively short period of time. Be prepared for it to take three to six years! The new facility must have certain "new" features, services or other attractions that their current facility currently does not have, to even raise a Specialist's interest. Having a new facility has its positive features if it has all the latest "bells and whistles" to make a specialists work easier, but that is only one component for their consideration.

There are many reasons doctors/specialists are careful about "joining" another facility where they will be required to purchase or lease an office/clinic to be in physical proximity of the hospital, either located within its premises, or a nearby Medical Office Building (MOB).

Let us briefly review a number of conditions and situations they will face.

52.1 For most doctors, any move other than across or down the same street may result in the doctor having to rebuild their practices (the further the distance the greater the rebuilding) all over, which could cause substantial financial issues for them, that will need to be addressed by the new hospital,

52.2 Existing patients typically prefer a doctor/specialist in the area near where they reside, as well as the fact different traffic patterns, or lack of public transport may cause them difficulty to go the new facility/clinic location, so they will become "lost patients" to the doctor's practice,

52.3 Issues relating to a new facility where the reputation as yet to be established, and where marketing of the facility's features, and services have to be promoted to create awareness, so there is risk in that aspect,

52.4 Location of clinic relative to hospital, transport accessibility, geographic and topological features,

52.5 Meeting the credentialing and certification requirements, e.g. "Board Certification", "Member of A Royal College in their Specialty", etc., of the new facility based on their set of Medical By-Laws,

52.6 Need to meet and develop a new internal referral network within the new hospital, which is dependent on a "critical" core of medical and surgical Specialists to complement their Specialty, and who meet their expectation of the clinical professional to justify referrals to them. It can be a "waiting game" for Specialists to move over, and can have impact on their personal financials pending resolution.

52.7 Developing new referral network of doctors in the community, which in many cases are difficult to re-establish and a powerful "pull" factor to remain, as many of them will go back to University time, and part of a good "old boy/girl" affiliation.

52.8 Need to develop new working relationships with Nurses, or encouraging some of the nurses to join them, as well as other professionals they trust and have a good working relationship,

52.9 Potential loss of affiliations with other Group Practices, Company Medical Panels of which they currently participate,

52.10 Being ostracized by fellow Specialists at their current facility once it becomes known they will be leaving, resulting in lack of internal referrals, and exclusion from internal activities and rosters.

In many instances recruitment of Doctors and Specialists from Institutional Practices, i.e. Public hospitals, University Hospitals, Military Facilities to private practice are the best candidates to "court" as they would be in the best position to migrate to the private sector. In any hospital, Government or Private, there must be a balance between senior, experienced Specialists, and new Specialists to provide depth of service, confidence and reputation, so this can present issues for both facilities with the Specialists caught "in the middle"

Further, in many countries Specialists from Government Hospitals are only allowed to work in the private sector on a part time basis, after completion of their scheduled times in the Government Hospital, so buildup of this group of Specialists will be slow. While in this "transition" phase, which can last years, it is common for very few Specialists to be in their private or hospital clinics in the mornings, with heavy workloads in the afternoons and evenings. In fact certain Specialists will want to avoid completely give up their relationship or appointment with the Government Hospital, as many are eligible for paid annual, sick, education/conference leave and other benefits which they will lose when they totally shift to private sector practice. However, once in the private sector and they have sufficiently grown their practices, Specialists can take on a Partner or make reciprocal arrangements with another Specialist to "attend to their patients" while they away. This can be done as often as they desire and can afford, so they just need to understand they will be "in charge" of their benefits, as opposed to being a recipient as an employee.

Just remember, these are all considerations when it comes time to set up a new facility and attracting Specialists to join the organization, so building up the workload and practice will take time. As in the opening statement, it is relatively easy to build a building, but very difficult to put the Medical Team together. Do not lose that perspective.

53 When setting up a new clinical service, there must be **a statistically suitable/acceptable number of good outcomes with high survival and success rate**, and low on complication and morbidity to establish

credibility for the service. This reflects directly on the Specialist.

For any new clinical service being started, or new Specialist joining and working in the Healthcare facility, there should be guidelines issued by the Medical Board on the minimum number of "basic" procedures performed to establish measurable, evidence based outcomes at the facility, before taking on more complex cases. Any hospital or new service is ultimately measured in three areas - Specialists skills, quality of the nursing, and quality of the related support services. So, any shortfall in these areas can have a negative effect on the outcome of the patient's condition, and ultimately, the success and reputation of the program.

When in discussion with the patient or family, a question that will inevitably arise is on the statistical percentage of "successful" outcomes (chance of survival), to give them comfort, and helping in their decision process, so it is important to perform sufficient number of procedures to be able to quote a reasonable success rate. The rationale is to ensure the Specialist, Nursing, and equipment are functioning "in harmony", comfortable with each other, and working as a coordinated Team. Each new Specialist given admitting and practice privileges should be subject to the same requirements, even if they have had outstanding outcomes at other facilities. Their clinical outcome rate at the Hospital or Healthcare facility will directly reflect on the reputation of both the Specialist and recognition of the Hospital as a provider, they are related!

As an example, a hospital decided to introduce a Cardiothoracic Service, and went out and recruited a Specialist, configured the OT/OR, purchased equipment, hired Nurses with cardio experience, and then commenced the program. The Medical Board gave directions that the Specialist must perform at least, a combined total of 100 basic Atrial Septal Defect (ASD), Ventricular Septal Defect (VSD) procedures, and various other procedures which would be closely monitored and reviewed before allowing him to take on more complex cases. The objective was to build up the survival rate percentage (statistic), so it could be shared that the Specialist had a 95-98% success rate for the patients on whom he operated. Patients, relatives, media, and others tend to look at the overall outcomes, and often make no distinction for very serious cases versus more basic cases so the success rate percentage rate is critical, and will "make or break" a new Specialist's reputation, program, as well as the image of the Hospital. For example, if a Specialist was not constrained and performed 10 cases which were a mix of basic and complex, and there were complications or negative outcomes (typically death or permanent physical deterioration within "x" number of days after the procedure) for five or six, then the success rate of the Specialist and Hospital would only be 40-50%! If another Specialist from another established facility (having performed hundreds or thousands of similar procedures) was under consideration and enjoyed a posted 93% success rate, which Specialist and Hospital would the patient and family be inclined to choose for their procedure? Therefore, it is critical to build up the success rate percentage, so when it comes time to perform more complex, risky procedures, should the Specialist "lose" a patient due to complexity or complications, the established success rate can still be managed and allow for selection of the Specialist and Hospital where a procedure will be performed. As Specialist's practice grows, then further detailed breakdowns on outcomes of specific types of high end treatment or surgical procedures can be provided by any Specialist in the Clinical Specialty. In some countries, names of the Specialist will even be published with their respective survival rates for comparison.

NOTE: Over time, Specialists will tend to become more expert in performing certain complex conditions and/or procedures, and gain a reputation amongst their peers, so other Specialists in the same specialty may refer their most complex/complicated patient cases to the "expert" Specialist to offer the best chance of success, even though the patient's condition has reached a stage where the success rate may still be low. Even though their success rate may be low, management by the expert Specialist may offer the best option available for the patient.

The number and types of procedures to be satisfactorily performed (meeting the acceptable statistical range) must be defined by the Medical Board for each particular Clinical discipline before the Specialists are credentialed to perform more complex cases. All Specialists must understand the principles and comply with the guidelines.

54   Design Hospitals and Healthcare Facilities to be patient Centric, and **ensure patient areas are functional and properly zoned** to contain activities, and avoid congestion.

As an Administrator, at some point in your career, you will be involved directly or indirectly in the design and/or layout of a Hospital or Healthcare facility. One of the key concepts to remember is proper grouping of patient functional services zones such as A&E/ER, Out-Patient Clinics, Ambulatory Day Treatment Services, In-Patient Admission Services, as well as Administrative support. All services should be designed for ease of access to Clinical Support Services such as, Imaging, Lab, and Pharmacy Services. Also be mindful of the various horizontal and vertical moving devices available to facilitate patient, visitor, staff, and vendor movement within and between zones of services. For more information on design and planning consideration, please avail yourself to "An Investor's Guide to Developing a Private Hospital – Ten Considerations before Committing" (Arthur Ouellette and Steven J Sobak) for the above type considerations as well and many others applicable ideas and concepts, whether for a new or redeveloped/renovated facility, private or public.

55 **Drugs administered in hospitals cost more** than purchasing similar items from the local Pharmacy for many reasons.

Often patients or caregivers will be very vocal about the costs of drugs and medications administered while an inpatient in a hospital, when they perceive they could go to a local pharmacy and with a prescription (or sometimes even without) purchase certain drugs and medications at a much lower cost.

The observation is correct, the cost of drugs and medications in a hospital setting is higher, but there are many factors that influence that cost which need to be taken into consideration, such as:

55.1 Purchase of the drugs and medications that meet the clinical standards, and evaluation of the best, and/or alternative options, to meet the medical requirement, e.g. "branded" vs "generic" for the patients. This is after evaluation, selection and approval of drugs and medications by the Hospital Drugs and Therapeutic Committee for inclusion as part of the facility's official Drug Formulary Listing,

55.2 Stocking and storing of sufficient inventory to be available 24 x 7 to meet the needs of the patients, regardless of when they come to hospital, considering long weekends, holidays. This includes monitoring of expiry dates, and taking actions to exchange or replace outdated drugs and medications with the drug companies,

55.3 Selecting, counting out the numbers of pills, caplets, measuring liquid medication for administration, packaging, and labeling for the patient, verifying the dosages are correct based on the age and/or weight of the patient, recording the manufacturing "lot numbers" and expiration dates of medications issued, as well as entering billing information into the computer system for inclusion on the patients bill, and updating the inventory records for the amount remaining,

55.4 Matching of the name of the medication against doctor's orders. Sometimes names of drugs and medications are very similar (but for different medical conditions) so care must be taken, and each prescription must be reviewed against of all other medications being taken or ordered to learn if there are any known contra-indications with others being taken at the same time, both Western and Traditional Chinese Medications (TCM), or has recently taken,

55.5 Transferring of the medications to the wards (manual or AGV), for distribution to the patients by the nurses or authorized nursing associates/aides, or pharmacists. Each individual administering the medications must verify the patient's name, hospital number, frequency, time, dosage, method of delivery, document administration, observe for any unexpected reactions or outcomes by the patient and documenting all this in the patient's medical record.

55.6 Certain provision for cost or loss of inventory due to limited life span of a medication, e.g. snake venom antidote, or return of the unused or outdated medications from patients/families which must be destroyed for safety reasons,

55.7 Insurance for liability of any untoward reactions, with the drugs,

55.8 Department local overhead, and an allocation for general overhead, and finally,

55.9 A financial contribution towards the operating margin of the organization.

For all these reasons, the cost of medication provided in a hospital or healthcare setting will be more expensive than the basic product one can purchase "off the shelf" in selected stores, or in a local pharmacy. A good analogy would be the purchase of raw food products from the market, preparing and eating the dish at home, versus eating the same dish in a hawker center, fast food center, or in a restaurant (open air, air conditioned etc.). Each will have a different pricing structure because of the labor involved in preparation, equipment required, location, ambiance, serving staff, general liability insurance, and in certain cases even the reputation of the Chef.

Understand what goes into the preparation and delivery of drugs and medications for each patient, and multiply this by the number of patients and frequency of dispensing throughout the day. Consider the total number of processes that are performed to ensure provision of the correct medication prescribed by the doctor, and safety of the patient.

56   Be prepared to address **questions about the high costs of healthcare**, as it is impossible to deny, but there are reasons and two powerful drivers, Cost and Usage. Let us start with exploring the Cost Driver.

There will always be individuals who will comment and raise issues about the high cost of seeking healthcare, often with remarks they are being "taken advantage of", lack of competition, etc. The reason of this perception is they are only looking at the end, and the fees and charges reflected on the Bill, without benefit of understanding the key components that build up the charges. There are **two main drivers for cost** of healthcare, actual Cost of providing healthcare in a structured facility, e.g. hospital, or other healthcare facility infrastructure and operating costs, and the Users of healthcare. This segment reflects on the cost aspect. Make sure you have a good understanding of the composition, and are confident, so you can explain it in a honest, open manner.

Manpower is by far the largest expense component and is represented by the Specialists and Nurses. While doctors comprise a relatively small number of FTEs, they are the most expensive resource as it is a function of their years of training and preparation. Depending on which country, Medical School and Residency training for between six to eight years to qualify for their basic Medical Degree and license to practice as a Physician (i.e., to work as a GP). Then another four to six years, sometimes more, to complete all their training to become a Specialist and therefore only by the time they are at least 30-35 years old are they capable to start an independent Specialist practice. So, even a small General Acute Hospital with 20 Admitting Specialists (FTEs), their cumulative education, training, and experience to treat patients could come to over 300 years (20 Specialists with an average of 15 years training) of collective experience available for the benefit of the patients! They are a precious resource. The more specialties provided by a Hospital, the greater this number. In most other industries and professions, by the time one reaches 30-35 years old, they would have been working for many years, and moved up the promotional ladder.

Nurses are the second largest manpower component in a hospital or healthcare facility, those with basic skills; all the way up through University Graduates with multiple degrees, and Specialty training as well to complement certain Specialists. They comprise the largest cohort of staff as the Nurses are required to look after patients on a 24 x 7 basis according to the patient's medical requirements. The Nurses are the individuals who carry out the instructions of the Doctors and Specialists, so are very important in ensuring patients receive their treatments and are regularly monitored.

Following the Nurses, there are many other professionals who have basic and advance degrees in order to meet the government requirements (Licenses), and Standards to meet local and international Accreditations in order to receive a Hospital License to open. In this group for example, are the Pharmacists, Laboratory Technicians, Therapist Professionals, and even Administrative staff with their degrees and certificates required to operate a Hospital. Operating expenses (OPEX) can be grouped into the following main categories.

56.1 Salaries, Benefits and Fees paid for required manpower comprises the largest component of a hospital budget, and in most years there is an inflation factor that must be addressed to retain staff so they are available when needed; hence annual increases.

56.2 Equipment. There are many pieces of expensive equipment in a hospital or healthcare facility that add costs but allows the professionals to perform their duties in diagnosis and treatment of the patients, such as MRI, CT, PET Scan, Angiography, General X-ray, Mammography, EEG, Echo, Laboratory Analyzing Consoles, Microscopes. From all the high tech equipment in the Operating Room/Theatre, Lasers, Linear Accelerator (LINAC), Robotics, multiple computer systems (hardware and software), server farms, and distributed computers within the facility, etc. to name a few.

56.3 Supplies, Consumables, and Implants used in treating of patients, as well as a wide variety of medications, that must be available to provide relief and infection management on a 24 x 7 day basis. Inventories.

56.4 Licensing, Regulations, Documentation requirements which all have a cost to implement and maintain, for the safety of the patient, and community.

56.5 Rental/Leases, Loans (major equipment) paid out to Government for use of facilities provided by the Government, or private Companies that built the facilities.

56.6 Building Maintenance Fees, Utilities, transportation vehicles, landscaping, etc.

56.7 Insurance for the buildings, vehicles, equipment, facility medical malpractice for staff, etc.

56.8 All these components are often "taken for granted" and invisible to the patient or family but must be available whenever an individual seeks medical help in a hospital or healthcare facility. With all the components in place and working, lives are saved, without it, outcomes could be less than satisfactory.

The combination of costs from the above examples of operating expenses makes healthcare provision high, as well as providing money for loan principle repayment and related interest payments used for construction and major infrastructure equipment acquisition, as well as dividends to shareholders for putting up money for the facility (in private hospitals), and providing working capital.

Very few industries are as complex as a hospital and/or healthcare facility. Hospitals and healthcare facilities have an obligation to keep costs under control, but so does the general public in using the various less expensive avenues to seek medical attention.

This description is simple, and less than complete but illustrates the key cost components associated with providing services in a hospital and all the resources required to make the hospital and/or healthcare facility a place where patients can receive basic and advanced medical treatment for most conditions; however, remember the old adage "nothing is for free". As the largest cost is manpower, every year "cost of living" adjustments will be made, which may result in adjustments.

So, it is impossible to deny hospital and healthcare costs are high, and will go up. What can be done is to ensure workloads are optimized, increases reflect external adjustments, are appropriate, and costs contained.

57   Be prepared to address **questions about the high costs of healthcare**, it is impossible to deny, but there are reasons. In this segment, let us explore the Usage Background that influences Hospital and Healthcare costs.

This part of the question of high healthcare costs relates to Usage and how it plays an important role in managing healthcare costs. Healthcare services are built on a pyramid shaped hierarchy of services.

57.1   Healthcare Education, Information, and Self Medication: This is the most basic care which must be promoted to make people aware of what can be self-treated, and when it is appropriate to seek professional medical care, e.g., headache, take aspirins obtained from a pharmacy, general cough and cold conditions, can also rest and self-medicate for basic symptoms, etc. This information should be learned from reading healthcare related bulletins, newspaper and magazine articles, internet searches, or previous experiences or interactions with doctors. This forms the base of the Healthcare Pyramid.

57.2 Primary Care: First level care services, comprised of single General Practitioner (GP-Physician) or multiple GP Clinics. General Practitioner Physician Doctors are those who focus on family medicine and are trained to treat a broad range of basic injuries and medical conditions, and who also access the patient to determine if they need to be referred to a Specialist, and if so, what Specialty. Primary care is also provided by Poly Clinics, Ambulatory Day Treatment Centers, Health Maintenance Organizations (HMOs), Company appointed Medical Panels, or equivalents, as well as, licensed Traditional or Chinese Medicine alternatives. Pediatricians and Geriatricians are Physicians who specialize looking after the myriad of conditions relating to children and the elderly.

57.3 Secondary Care: General Acute Hospitals staffed by Specialists, but may not provide full range of Specialists in all medical specialties, or able to treat the more/most complex medical conditions. Acute Rehabilitation Hospitals are generally considered Secondary Care facilities. Most patients are managed at this level.

57.4 Tertiary Care: General Acute Hospitals that provide a wider range of Medical Specialties, and sub-Specialties for treatment by experienced Specialists, or Specialty Centers with sub-Specialties, e.g. Eye, Heart (Cardiac), Neurology/Neurosurgery, Obstetric, Oncology, Orthopedic, Pediatric, Skin, etc., most surgical procedures are performed at Hospitals in this Category of Care group, and finally,

57.5 Quaternary Care: Similar and related to Tertiary Hospital and Specialty Center facilities but with the highest end equipment (e.g., Linear Accelerator, PET Scan) and treatment modalities (research, and certain "cutting edge" procedures) for most complex medical conditions. Basically if the condition cannot be treated at this level of Hospital or Specialty Center, then there are most likely, no other medical or surgical options available. Certain Departments in a Tertiary Level Hospital can provide Quaternary Level services, and these Hospitals, Centers, Departments are considered the top/apex of the Pyramid.

However, for patients who receive medical services in countries with "no out of pocket", low fee payment schemes; or, patients enrolled in "first dollar" medical insurance coverage schemes, they tend to choose the more expensive alternatives, since there is a perception of "no cost to them", leading to overconsumption and inappropriate use of higher end services. Further, there is another large cohort of healthcare seekers with the mentality/perception to "bypass" the valuable GP level services and "go straight to the top, to the Best" to shortcut the process, even before they have yet to define their medical condition which then determines the Medical Specialty of Specialist who needs to be consulted!

For proper use of the healthcare system, patients should follow the treatment hierarchy outlined above. At each level above primary care, more tests and procedures will need to be performed to analyze the patient's condition which will add costs related to the treatment. Only after an assessment by a GP-Physician/Specialist should any decision be taken to arrange for an appointment with a specific Secondary Care Level Medical Specialist, if necessary.

Unfortunately many patients choose to enter the healthcare system at the Secondary or Tertiary Care Levels, so they consume more services, tend to overload the system resulting in longer waiting and scheduling times, which in turn increases their costs, and bill size. Therefore, as stated in the beginning, healthcare consumers play a major role as contributors to rising healthcare costs, and can help contain costs by utilizing the system properly. As Administrators, we must educate the public.

58 **Service Quality is a mindset**, something that must be developed, nurtured, and practiced in order to become inculcated in the way we deliver our service.

This observation is now a common theme for many motivational and service quality consultants and speakers who sponsor programs and seminars with this theme; however, it has yet to be universally adopted, so the initial observation is still relevant.

Basically it is a situation whereby the work performed whether directly on or for patients or indirect role, the work should be of the highest quality given the resources available. Service quality is comprised of at least two components, the "hard" component which is the actual physical products or services we sell, and the "soft" component which is the human element. Combined they set the standards of quality delivered to the patient.

The "hard" component represents all the medical supplies, consumables, pharmaceutical items, as well as the equipment used in treating and delivering the service. Quality of these items should be commensurate with the budget available and achieving the best quality and outcome possible. This requires staff to select the most appropriate items, ensure they are of design, composition, and construction that is safe for the patient, and of the highest ethical standards, i.e. no imitation, or counterfeit ingredients or components that could negatively affect the clinical and medical outcome of the patients. So staff must take responsibility to ensure they evaluate, and select the items within their budget, yet meets their clinical specifications, and remove from service any items identified as failing to meet operating standards and set aside for repair or replacement.

The "soft" component is the human element. At times managing the "hard" component is easier than the soft, as creating a sense of responsibility and understanding their contribution of providing services to the best of their abilities can at times be lacking. The correct attitude requires staff to segregate their personal issues from their duties at work. This is easier said than done, but staff must make the conscious effort, lest they become "lazy" (even for a short time) and take shortcuts that could negatively impact the treatment of the patient. All staff have an obligation to do their best in provision of service, so awareness and attitude must be fostered and constantly nurtured. Staff should avoid being self-conscious of their roles or positions within the organization. Each staff and position in the organization is there for a purpose. If it is not required, it should be eliminated. So each staff should feel committed.

For example, housekeeping/environmental staff often believed their roles were so menial that other staff, and even patients, looked down on them since they are frequently some of the least educated, most senior in age, and were "invisible" as they went about their work. Only after considerable time was invested to educate them and change to a new paradigm, one where they learned they contributed and had an important role in keeping the patient rooms and areas clean, linens changed, toilets sanitized and presentable, as they often spent more time with patients than either the nurses or doctors and they created a pleasant environment for the patients did they begin to understand the importance their roles. So by developing their service quality mindset, and raising their self-esteem they, were taught the importance of proper care in their appearance (such as clean, tidy, ironed uniforms, wearing of some make-up, selected jewelry pieces), and encouraged to make "small talk" with the patients such that they took pride in their work, confidence improved, and they identified and took ownership with the quality of their work. The service quality mentality finally became part of their culture, and they started receiving more compliments than they ever had previously. Environmental staff were also provided with checklists of tasks to be performed in each type room (suite, deluxe, single, double, four, six bedded), along with photos of properly cleaned rooms and layout to assist them. While housekeeping/environmental staff was used in this example, the same principles of understanding and approaches should be shared with any medical, nursing or other professional junior staff in training, aides, assistants, even personnel, and finance "back room" administrative and facility staff (e.g. wearing of gloves when removing/replacing ceiling tiles to avoid dirty finger and hand prints) to take care of the details to minimize repeat of 'non value add" (washing and removing prints) work. Needless to say, the senior staff must also be oriented and trained to adopt the same mindset to lead by example and promote Service Quality expectations.

These examples are simple, but illustrate the need to combine the hard and soft components of Service Quality and inculcate a mindset in all staff regardless of their role, to make the patient's journey and experience in the healthcare facility the best it can be.

59 Whenever staff of an organization are to be recognized or rewarded (monetarily, certificates/plaques, name list) for any special reason, e.g. SARS, participating in helping in a disaster situation, **remember to include the staff who are part of contractual/ business partners who also participated. They are/were part of your Team.**

Never forget that everyone in the organization contributes to the protection and well-being of the patients, and should be recognized and treated as if they were "on payroll" of the organization. Remember, the use of contractual outsourcing services and developing service "partnerships" with management are "tools" and used to achieve results in specific areas with staff specially trained, but could be converted back to "payroll staff" under certain conditions. The point of this comment is that whenever the entire organization is mobilized to address an emergency (whether national or organizational in scope) all staff available are included, and engaged. So, when the crisis or emergency is over, all staff, both payroll based and contractual/partnership should be treated and recognized as ONE TEAM for coming together in a time of need. If any special efforts are being considered to recognize all staff, outstanding individuals, or Teams, with certificates, or other mementoes, this should be done regardless of the underlying employment arrangement, they are your staff. Even if the Board or other supporting organizations want to allocate certain funding for bonuses, or small "tokens of appreciations" such as "ang pows/red packets" or shopping coupons, remember that the contractual/partnership, and even volunteer staff, should be included. Most likely the contractual and partnership budgets did not make provision to absorb all the increased costs, such as overtime, or illness, incurred during the crisis or emergency, so any incremental amount that can also be shared amongst their staff would also be appropriate and appreciated for their participation and support, as most likely, their Company Service Contracts/Agreements did not include budgetary provisions for this magnitude of disruption. By including all staff, this promotes unity, cohesiveness, and morale.

60   The best way to learn about a surgical Specialist's suitability and temperament is to **ask the OT Nurse Managers at facilities where they work/worked**, as they are the ones who have to hold the

Teams together and have the "inside" story on their behavior.

This was an ingenious method to learn more about surgical Specialists, and their ability to interact with other members of the Surgical Team, specifically other Specialists, OR/OT Nurses, and Therapists, e.g. Perfusionist. While many surgical Specialists are very technically skilled, the pressure and responsibility is substantial, yet they also need to be professional and civil to the nurses, and other staff in the Operating Rooms/Theatres.

If any particular Specialist becomes easily agitated, very physical, throwing instruments, implants and supplies around, or being verbally loud, abusive, insulting, or condescending to the Nurses and supporting staff, the tension will be very high, and lead often time generate low morale, often time to the point where the Nurses want to be reassigned, or even resign as the atmosphere is "toxic" and this could affect their concentration, putting patients at risk.

It was one of the Chief/Head Nursing Officer who shared this "suggestion" to obtain the real information about the mannerisms of a Specialist and their attitudes in the Operating Room, and that is to contact the OR/OT Head Surgical Nurse at previous hospitals where the surgical Specialist previously worked, as it is ultimately the Head Nurse's responsibility to develop and retain the necessary number of Nursing Teams to support the surgical Specialists.

So in addition to the usual background checks performed by the Human Resource staff and Specialist peer references, a reference request could be made to engage the Senior Nursing staff to make contact with the Senior Surgical Nurses from other previous facilities to secure feedback on the Specialists. If done correctly and in a tactful manner, obtaining a proper assessment will save the organization time in the long run by engaging Specialists who can work as part of the Team. This information can be shared with the Hospital's Senior Medical Staff making the final hiring decisions, so they will be able to ensure the best Specialists are engaged, and also preserve their Nurses.

61 **Many staff positions** within a healthcare facility **can be filled by individuals who have a physical disability**, so make sure office, and back room areas have toilets, rest areas built or modified to accommodate the staff, and ensure access to the areas also designed barrier free.

Most healthcare facilities now make efforts to ensure there is "barrier free" access designed to accommodate handicapped/challenged public, and patients; however, one area often overlooked are similar facilities for the organization's own staff, in the internal working areas of the healthcare facility.

Depending on the position description requirements, Managers should be hiring staff based on the applicant's mental abilities, attitude and skills to complete the defined tasks, as well as having the necessary physical mobility attributes to perform. For example, wheelchair dependent staff in a Call Center, Communications/Telephone Operators, Accounting/Finance, Human Resource, Information Technology Departments,

Legal, Customer Service, or Media Management, etc., are typically considered "back room/back of the house" type services where staff can have certain physical mobility disabilities, yet are capable to perform the tasks required. Therefore, design arrangements should be taken into consideration to ensure certain staff toilets, staff eating/rest areas, meeting rooms, even office entrances, staff lifts, desks are designed to allow access by individuals using a wheelchair, walker, or other devices to ambulate. Architects should apply design specifications, e.g. access to toilets, similar for the physically disabled in both office, and back room areas as for the public areas.

A good way to determine if your facility has been designed adequately to cater for handicapped staff is to engage one or more staff who are wheelchair bound, or friends in wheelchairs to visit the facility, starting with the car parking and drop off points to conduct a survey, and highlight all areas and obstacles where they encountered difficulty in moving around.

Hiring disabled staff allows them to contribute in a positive manner to the healthcare support community, as well as the specific healthcare facility taking their abilities seriously. Not surprisingly, they also become very loyal employees of the organization, thankful for giving them the opportunity to work productively according to their education and skills!

62   In the private sector, **Specialists** affiliated with a Hospital or Healthcare Facility **can often provide names of fellow Specialists** who may be interested and willing to join a new facility.

Many times in the private sector, Specialists who have already joined a Hospital or Healthcare facility are one of the best individuals for identifying other Specialists, from the same specialty or another who may be interested in joining. They tend to know who may be "in the market", interested in or considering leaving for another practice, either in the Public or Private sector, and who they are comfortable working with and referring patients. Most Specialists know their colleagues in the same medical Specialty via meetings, Specialty Conference, working together, going all the way back to Medical School and various postings during training. Often time they are willing to provide names, and/or even an introduction to the Administrator (CEO or CMB) to follow up for consideration. If approved, they can submit their assessments of the candidate's CVs to the Medical Staff Evaluation and Selection Committee. Leading up to this point, there will most likely be one or more interview sessions to share relevant information and become comfortable with the prospects. These meetings normally occur after normal work hours, and around the dining table. They can either be as a one-on-one session, or including the spouse (or significant other) as the opportunity becomes more encouraging. It is important to ensure the significant other is also included, at least on a social basis so they have an opportunity to meet, understand the challenges, and ask questions (schools for children, religious service, employment prospects, shopping, social aspects, etc.) since acceptance of the position would have material impact on the entire family. Once all aspects are reviewed, and cleared by the Evaluation Committee, an offer can be made to the Specialist for direct employment on payroll, or granting Admitting Privileges to independent Specialists affiliated with the Hospital or

Healthcare facility, depending on the Practice Model followed. There may be many variants in the "terms of engagement" for consideration.

So, if new medical staff are recruited in this manner and join the organization, this will allow for a more seamless integration of individuals, and services which will develop and enhance the internal referral network.

OPERATIONAL RELATED OBSERVATIONS

1 Always **WRITE FROM THE READER'S PERSPECTIVE.** Never presume the reader has the same level of understanding or background as you, the writer. Always have someone, not familiar with the topic, read your letter/document before sending it out to determine if the responses are clear and the points/questions raised are answered.

This observation could relate to any industry; however healthcare offers a particularly interesting challenge since the environment is constantly evolving so terminology and background context to any response must be clarified. When someone writes in to the healthcare facility, whether as complaint, or just seeking clarification of process or procedure, the writer/responder should structure the response using words the reader can understand. Make efforts to provide background context, or offer definitions to terminology and abbreviation used to convey an explanation where necessary, while ensuring the basic question(s) or issue(s) are being addressed.

"Jargon" refers to terms used in a specific industry, and healthcare has over the years built up a substantial inventory of words which have meaning to individuals in the healthcare industry, but are confusing or have little context to most "lay people" outside the industry. Another good example is what people refer to as "legalese", all the terms and specific writings is certain formats which are understandable by those in the legal profession, but create barriers to those outside the profession. The same happens within the healthcare environment. For this reason, it is recommended the respondent have individuals who are independent of the question asked, or in crafting responses, read both components and determine if they understand the question and the response is clear and understandable. Any confusion indicates the response needs to be revised. The independent party can be other staff, your boss, or even a family member (depending on confidentiality), and they should be "tasked" with the request to answer "does the crafted response make sense and answer the question(s) raised?" Only a "yes" response is acceptable. For any other response, seek further clarification of the points, and make additional revisions to the response. Then ask another independent party to read! If the basic question being raised lacks clarity, it may be appropriate to make telephone contact to clarify the question(s). Failure to do so will result in further "rounds" of communications, and each becoming more expensive in time to resolve.

This principle should also be followed within the organization, as staff may have other perceptions, and in some instances the same terminology or abbreviations may have different meaning. So someone in Finance needs to be sensitive to clinical, research, or other staff in the facility to ensure the terms are clarified as required. Within the facility, if there is any question, it is more convenient to make telephone contact. When responding to the Ministry or other Governmental Body, also ensure the explanations are clear. At the end of any communication, always close with the name of a Contact person, telephone number, and email address to facilitate if there are still any questions.

2   For planning purposes, always remember - **The more complex the question, the shorter the response time given.**

This typically happens when Boards or Director/Trustees, various Government Bodies meet and information discussed leads to issues requiring further clarification, analysis, projections, details, etc. Members of the high level meetings will want to resolve their concerns before taking decision or actions, so giving due respect to the Source of the questions, extraordinary efforts need to be taken, which includes engaging Managers from multiple Departments to either be "on call" or help gather data and/or perform required actions to answer the queries. A good example would be where Members of the Board want additional assumptions to be taken into consideration, requiring future population projections and disease indices, and then generating alternative pro-forma(s) to answer their immediate concerns. Gathering and generating the responses may involve a number of staff, and even require overnight work in order to prepare an appropriate response to the Board. Further, efforts needs to be taken to anticipate potential questions that could even emerge from the data provided, and have it available should the need require.

Remember, members of the high level Meetings are strategic thinkers and planners who may be privy to information not readily available, and they are usually looking at the "larger picture", so their questions are usually quite complex. They want data to determine if their information is correct (validation) or want to know the potential impact should certain events "come to pass". Most Board Meetings are held, late morning, afternoon, or evenings, so this leaves a short window for response, and requires quickly mobilizing necessary individuals who can provide the information. At times we have had responses come in late Friday, and requiring a response by Monday (the next official workday), the weekend/holiday/leave plans may be need to be modified or sacrificed. Often time it is the IT Department, Finance, Operations and Legal Departments most heavily impacted. A good practice is to announce the major meetings being held and place all key Department Heads "on call" during or after the meeting to minimize response time.

This type of situation also occurs when there is a major breach in confidentiality of information, or a real/perceived shortfall in medical care leading individuals to approach various Ministries, or Media to seek answers. Once this occurs, questions will be raised, and staff must be mobilized to provide preliminary, interim, and final answers to manage the situations. Again, in these instances the questions raised are both normally complex and time sensitive, so necessary staff must be mobilized from CEO/MD down to address the individuals raising the issues, as well as the Ministries and Media, so this will require substantial efforts by the various Departments, particularly Corporate Communications typically responsible as the "public face" of the organization as well as, Clinical, Legal and Operations Departments.

3   When requesting information, **always share the background on the intended use**, so the information provided will meet the requirements, and preclude embarrassment. Conversely, the potential provider/source individual of any requested information should ask for the background, before blindly proceeding to provide the data, and avoid double work.

How a request for information is asked, will determine the type of information provided. Therefore, whenever I ask for information to be gathered, I try to provide a brief background and context on where the information will be shared, and how it will be used, and if there are any special considerations to be factored in the response. Further, I will ask if there are any questions on the instructions provided for the purpose of minimizing any misunderstanding. Without clarification the information provided can be correct in a general manner, but be incomplete, or worse still, misrepresenting the facts when compared with submissions from other entities when combined and presented as results of a survey, or in a chart causing incorrect conclusions to be drawn and decisions taken.

A simple example that has occurred on various occasions is the answer to the "simple" question "what is the average salary of XYZ professional position"? Without explanation of what the purpose of the question is, or understanding how the person making the requests plans use it, the range of answers reported will range from the basic monthly/annual average salary, to a complete compensation package. In fact, if the intention is to convey a comprehensive compensation profile for a position(s) remuneration package, content of compensation package should be further refined to include such components as the value of annual, holiday, sick, family, conference/seminar leave, medical/life/accidental death, med-mal and other insurance premiums, bonuses, regular overtime payment, and "benefits in kind", etc. To add another complicating dimension, at times the requests come from a higher level such as Corporate HQ, or a Department/Ministry, passed through one or two layers of Human Resource Departments for collection. Without proper clarification and context, when the paper, document, or media article is completed and distributed, the graphs and tables will display a substantial range. Depending on the purpose for gathering the information, the "target" audience can draw incorrect conclusions and make decisions based on "skewed" data with results that can be quite confusing and detrimental to certain facilities, and even individuals, reporting more or less information than what was intended or required.

I would tell my staff if they "blindly" prepare information without knowing how it is to be used, I will hold them accountable, and they may need to rework/redo the information, if there is time, and this is all "no value-add" activity. Regardless of the requesting source, as supervisors and managers, we must inculcate staff to take the initiative to ask questions to ensure before investing valuable time and effort to collect the data, they understand the purpose and requirement. Further, they should not be intimidated by the answer that "Corporate/Board/Minister" so-and-so is requesting the data – what data!! If and staff is not comfortable with questioning the requesting individuals, raise it to the attention of their most senior staff, so they may seek clarification. In principle, understanding the end purpose for the use of the information whether it is for financial, operational, or clinical information is critical. Poor or incorrect information will also reflect negatively on the higher level staff, so they have a vested interest to ensure accuracy.

4   Always take time to read and understand the content of any document you sign. **Once signed, you "own it", and will be "responsible" for any outcome, good or bad.** Professionally dangerous to assume

that someone who signs before you did their "due diligence", so do not sign "blindly".

This is a very important concept that is frequently overlooked and can have severe repercussions, all the way from counselling to termination and/or legal action. While many individuals are extremely busy, such as doctors, nurses, administrators, with many documents requiring their signatures, they must take sufficient time to read documents before signing, since once signed it conveys that it is correct and reflects the professional's position. While subordinates, secretaries, assistants, peers in other roles within the organization may help in preparation, reading, or vetting of documents, agreements or statements, it is still the signor who takes ultimate responsibility and ownership for the content. Trust is great (as in confidence in the person who completed the document pending your signature), but one's reputation and livelihood depends on the accuracy, correctness, and completeness of the documents, so it is imperative you read before signing. To request return of a signed document for modification or replacement after signing projects a lack of thoroughness and carelessness in one's work process and system, which by extension, could suggest the professional services provided may not be of appropriate standard. Further, other actions and decisions may result from documents provided; for example, a Senior Administrator must declare all the medical services provided at a hospital, clinic, or other facility for professional liability insurance. If new clinical services (perhaps considered high risk) were added at the facility, yet omitted on the insurance declaration document at submission, and something untoward happened while performing a procedure of treatment using one of the new services and a claim for negligence or damages is made, oversight in ensuring completeness of the document disclosure content could result in denial of part or all insurance coverage, resulting in personal or organizational exposure of the financial shortfall to address the incident. There are also incidents where a junior staff completed the correct information for an insurance claim report, but mixed-up two patients, and the doctor signed both forms without reading them completely resulting in delay in settlement of the insurance, and embarrassing all the individuals involved. Most entities, depending on the value or responsibility of the undertaking have an organizational hierarchy requiring multiple signatories to indicate relevant staff have reviewed the work, from lower to more senior, so work responsibly.

The message is, in most instances it takes only a few seconds, minutes to review every document before you sign, to ensure it is correct and complete as it will reflect on your professionalism, and avoiding all the "no value-added" costs incurred to rectify any problems created. Obviously the higher up the organizational hierarchy the signor is, the greater the consequences will be, should the document information be incorrect.

5 Remember, **every decision taken** has a financial/tax, legal, and potentially IT implication, so share accordingly, and obtain necessary input.

Just a reminder that within the organization whatever we do, whatever decision taken has a financial impact. It either increases, reduces, or "breaks-even" within or between departments experiencing the impact. Further many decisions have tax or governmental implications, e.g. privacy, disclosure, monopoly or oligopoly, etc., which need to be considered, and finally, with all the computerization, there will be IT implications, i.e. software, hardware, manpower requirements for installation, development/testing, security, and finally implementation. These are all "hurdles/obstacles" that must be cleared. Then, only after the net positive/negative impact, as determined by an incremental pro-forma preparation, will management be in the position to render a "final" decision. Prior to the complete analysis, the status of the decision should be regarded as an "in-principle" approval until all the "green lights" have been achieved, and hurdles cleared.

Sometimes individuals become excited over possibilities without assessing the key Enterprise Risk Management elements that can impact the outcome. Individuals without sensitivity or exposure to financial analysis can overlook this process, so it should be mandatory for individuals in Supervisory, Managerial be given training (by the CFO/FC) or obtain formal instructions on cost and risk management to create the decision awareness process. This learning point will become critical to all Senior Management and should be part of their professional development over the years, if they have aspirations to move up in the organizational hierarchy, or even remain in the present positions.

With proper training, the staff will automatically perform this type or review prior to presentation or seeking approval of any material changes.

6   As Administrators and Financial professionals, it is important to take time to **visit the "frontlines" to observe what and how procedures are performed.**

Observe different types of surgeries, e.g. "open heart" in an OT, delivery of a baby, MRI or CT Scan being administered, and as many of the hundreds of other procedures performed in a hospital or medical facility as possible. Walk the Wards, oversee therapies being provided, be "attached", to learn how Departments/Services function. Basically, **learn the details on how services are delivered**, so you can relate and make better decisions when support is requested, or new/replacement equipment is requested.

Over the years we find that many administrators and financial staff have little understanding of the medical services being performed in the hospital, and this is an embarrassing situation. In order to be a good administrator or financial individual it is incumbent that time is taken to learn about procedures, what equipment is required, supplies used, and staff required so there is a better understanding on the part of the administrators and finance people to understand and appreciate requests from the clinical and medical staff to complete their tasks. When I started out in healthcare, I was placed on a one year rotation to different Departments within the hospital to gain exposure to the work performed. So, I spent time attached to the Nursing Department, Pharmacy, as well as Housekeeping/Environmental, and Facilities Departments. For the duration of each attachment, I was used to perform routine tasks under supervision of the professionals. Later I took the personal initiative to meet with surgeons to obtain permission to observe various surgeries, such as open heart, and neuro surgeries so I could better relate to the procedures and requirements. As a result I became much more aware of the clinical and nursing services, and other department requirements, so was more understanding and appreciative of their requirements and responsibilities. A good "by-product" of showing interest, it allowed for development of good working relationships with all the individuals, and built trust and understanding.

While it is unfortunate that the attachment practice/concept is very seldom practiced anymore, particularly over a period of a year, a shorter version could perhaps be designed for senior staff of a certain level. This learning process should be extended to the wards and other treatment areas to observe and learn about how services are delivered.

7   Many times we do **"The Same Thing, ONLY Different"**.

In management operations and strategic thinking there are many ideas and approaches to address problems and issues. Times change, organizations evolve, older staff are replaced by new, and latest generation staff who have different work profiles, attitudes, tolerances, and expectations. Over time, ideas and strategies are reviewed and presented in new formats with new terms/terminology, approaches, most likely supplemented with current technology to make sharing of ideas and implementation acceptable in a jargon understood by current management. However, the reality of the situation, perceptions, and in some instances refinement of initiatives resulting in a "repackaging" of previous actions but taken to another level of understanding. In any business the key drivers requiring management are revenue, expenses, workload and productivity, alignment and interactions to optimize resources, attention to regulatory and legal compliance, and leveraging on IT to achieve better performance. Senior Management must function as an "orchestra conductor" who decides on the objectives to be achieved and "tweak" the various "instruments" in the organization to achieve objectives via the tools and methodologies available.

Only when a paradigm shift occurs in terms on the way services are delivered can there be real change. This is dependent both on technology (IT, technology innovation) and a culture where staff keep an "open mind" to new ideas that will change the approach, yet achieve the traditional goals of keeping the organization viable, using metrics that are understandable and measurable.

8   Stay around long enough, and you will observe **the same rationale used 20-30 years ago, to justify proposed changes to the current structures and processes**, being used, in all or part, to revert back to the previous configuration, e.g., centralized to decentralized, to centralized functions and vice versa.

Over the years this "phenomenon" has occurred in various organizations. We have had the opportunity to join a couple organizations shortly after a major infrastructure decision change occurred and was being implemented, and have also been a participant in several more changes. The change could represent a complete 180° reversion involving the entire organization, or only certain components; brought about by a modification to the old concept, but typically driven by access to new technology or Board strategy; however, the outcome is that the basic organizational infrastructure has been substantially modified. At times, service departments, or service provision functions can even result in being "spun off" to create new companies/entities.

Typical examples of rationale and explanations often used for proposed changes going in either direction. It will –

8.1 Allow for less bureaucracy, and improves response time,
8.2 Give more autonomy to the Business Entities to promote healthy competition (professional, operational, pricing, and financial),
8.3 Reduce duplication in work effort,
8.4 Ease in Consolidation or elimination of redundant functions to create more efficiency,
8.5 Allow for reduction of the Corporate Overhead, and manpower,
8.6 Ensure decisions are more representative of the of the geographic area being served,
8.7 Dismantle "silo" mentality(ies), to ensure better harmony and coordination between Headquarters and Facilities,
8.8 Standardize operation and achieve "economy of scale",
8.9 Take advantage of certain legal requirements for the benefit of the organization,
8.10 Improve management, and talent development for succession planning.

Normally after a number of years, shortcomings will be identified within the current system, and perceived that a change in structure is required, often leading to a operational model similar to one from 20-30 years ago. New generation management philosophies emerge, IT and other technology continues to improve, new Government policies and regulations are implemented, corporate governance practices and enforcement are often the key "drivers" which lead to strategic decisions on whether to adopt "new" approaches, often unaware of the previous history. The irony is when the changes require shareholdings, i.e. consolidations, divesting, new companies, etc., it is the lawyers who benefit most from the process, and creates a large financial hurdle for the organization to overcome.

This observation is to share and create awareness. Change is inevitable, and healthcare business goes in cycles, and circles following the latest concepts, hopefully each time for the better. The benefit of these constant changes is that work will be created, money infused into the industry/economy, and people gainfully employed, with sets of skills, a newer generation!

9 Remember, **there are no "second chances"** when trusted individuals intentionally release sensitive payroll, patient, or confidential operational information. The trust is lost, the staff is released.

This is a sensitive topic, so all staff upon being hired, must be instructed on the importance of compliance and the related consequences for non-compliance. Further, staff should also be informally reminded periodically to reinforce the need for compliance, and formally, at least annually on the importance of compliance. As Managers, Supervisors, Directors, trust is automatically extended to all individuals hired and working within the department or organization. From an operational perspective this is the position I have taken over the years in all departments reporting directly or indirectly to me in all my senior position as CEO, COO, or CFO. Staff in certain Departments such as Finance, Human Resources, and Material Management (Purchasing), and Medical Records all handle and manage sensitive documents with information classified as "confidential" or higher. Other departments need to identify the confidential information and processes that also require special attention. If any staff is in doubt, they should take a position the information is confidential while they clarify or seek clearance before releasing information to protect both themselves and the organization.

Should any confidential or higher level classified information be released without proper authorization by an empowered individual, the fate of the staff involved will result in termination. Depending on the impact of the released information, both civil and criminal action, in addition to termination could be initiated by the organization for damages, or individuals whose privacy has been violated. The only exceptions to this policy has been when complying to conditions of an approved "whistleblowers" law.

Introduction of Personal Data Protection laws in many countries further enforces the sensitivity about release of confidential or protected information/data, and makes penalties applicable to the organization and Data Protection Officer quite substantial.

10. Should I pass away quickly from a massive stroke or heart attack, when trying to establish "cause of death", do not first look at money, or women. **Look to the computer**, as it causes so much stress when it fails to operate correctly, perform the basic functions, or tries to do more than you require, e.g., correct spelling but substituting a completely different word which changes the context.

While this appears to be a "lighthearted" comment, there is actually more substance to it than what may appear on the surface. While we have been using computers at work, and home since they first emerged as a tool, it is becoming more difficult to keep up with all the versions, improvements, and new built in features, that try to make the software "smarter" such as spelling, and grammar fixes. In that process, so many new features have been added to the software it is difficult to learn them and what activates the feature, and often only learn of a feature when we "hit a wrong key" and the program shifts into other modes with which we are not familiar, or the program wants, or makes unwanted changes. In the effort to salvage the situation and return to where we were before all the new features took over, we become more confused and frustrated, and particularly so when it appears that we have lost part or all of a file we have diligently been working on for a period of time. We recognize that we need to regularly save our information, but there are times when we get so caught up with what we are doing, and the information is readily flowing that we overlook the saving part until something happens. At that time the frustration and stress level escalates to a point where we want to "change the physical configuration" of the computer and software. As we spend so much time on the computer, it has become the "mistress" of our life, so I tell my wife if she ever receives a call from work that something ever happened to me, such as a heart attack or stroke, the likely culprit will be the computer, and not another woman, or money. No need to look further!

As much of my time at the office is on the office computer, and many nights and weekends at home, to have a file "lost or damaged", is very demoralizing. I find that I normally am so drained after such an episode that I cannot get myself motivated to start the process over for a period of time, and usually end up waiting till the next day to start all over. But even then, the reconstructed files may not contain or reflect the energy and passion that was in the lost file.

The computer frustration also extends to the various devices connected to the computer. Why does the printer's features, e.g. scan, copy, fax, not work today when used only recently, and they worked? We then spend valuable time trying to troubleshoot the problem on what, or how it changed. Oftentimes the only solution is to reset the program, and we "hold our breath" hoping all the settings are retained; however, if not we must then reset them.

When this happens at work, we do have the benefit of contacting our IT staff who come to the rescue. They complete the recovery task in short time and probably wonder "what is the matter with us"! At home, the ready fix is the children, grandchildren, or neighbor's children who appear to have the "magic touch" to resolve the problem, and they usually leave me wondering "what is the matter with me"?

For all the above reasons, I find computers and related devices that are supposed to our make lives and work easier, create more challenging and stressful situations when they fail to work as programmed. As a result, they create unnecessary stress because we have become so dependent on them. The key thing I have learned over the years is to save and back-up your files. Sometimes that works!!

11   **Auditors (both internal and external) are "trained and educated" by the organization** about the business they are auditing, and then charge the organization a fee for the privilege of learning the business, and telling them all the areas that need improvement.

This is an observation made over the years whenever Auditors, either internal or external, are engaged to perform their annual financial reviews. During the first year, the financial management team, CFO, FC, and other Senior Managers, spend considerable time working with the new Auditors to educate them on operations and working within the hospital or healthcare facility. Part of the time is expended to explain the history of various accounts, standards, and terminology/jargon used in the industry. This is the organization's investment in the Auditors. The Auditor's take this knowledge back and use it to form their knowledge base for developing their respective Audit approach, schedules, and reviews to be conducted.

Apart from the basics learned, the Auditors use the information shared with them to "add value" by developing various "benchmarks" whereby they begin measuring our financial and operational performance (depending on the scope) making suggestions on how to improve our processes and operations particularly relating to the financial aspects. In many instances they look to "best practices" of other industries with the objective to transfer selected practices from them to the hospital or healthcare setting. After all the training and orientation by the facilities, the Auditor's then share various points via the Management Letter to the Board and Senior Management.

However, when Auditors are engaged with healthcare experience, the time spent for orientation is much less, and normally the Audit Fees are priced lower, than those where they must "learn the business". Their Fees are then more dependent on the quality of the financial state of affairs, and the amount of work to understand them so as to render an "opinion".

12   Remember Auditors, through their random or selective sample size selection, **will always find the one document/incident** you wish would remain buried.

As part of annual financial audits, the Auditing Firm/Company engaged will perform "tests" of your systems to determine if the processes are working correctly, and the interests of the organization are being served. For that, they will identify and select a number of transactions often stratified by value for their inspections. Various algorithms are used to select documents but in that selection process they will identify a document(s) that requires explanation. Sometimes a series of transactions are really questionable in nature and will lead to expansion of their review sample which could potentially identify an endemic problem with potentially serious consequences. These aberrations may need to be brought up the highest levels (Senior Management and/or Board) for information and action. In other instances the documents (or lack of) are not ideal, but still sufficient to justify the transaction was legitimate, but none-the-less potentially embarrassing, and requiring additional explanations and proof to clarify the situation and circumstances. As an example, the support document for payment for certain goods may be lacking the original "Delivery Receipt", lost/misfiled for some reason. To clear the outstanding payment, Finance, may request a "certified true" copy of the Delivery document from the vendor, and the Hospitals receiving staff must inspect and trace the delivery to internal storage or delivery. Other situations can arise around Contracts and Agreements without clearly defined "deliverables", resulting in further clarification to ensure payments are correct.

This review can occur in any Departments where documentation must be maintained in proper order, such as the obvious, Finance, but also includes:

12.1 Human Resources with regards to documents supporting the hiring and termination processes, reference checks, Letters of Offers, validation of education certificates, insurances, previous employment, etc.;

12.2 Material Management, with regards to proper purchasing of supplies, materials, services following proper quote or tender/bidding requirements based on the total value/cost of items and ensuring non-splitting of Purchase Orders to circumvent required hierarchy approval;

12.3 Pharmacy Department, in capturing and recording quantity of drugs and supplies provided. Often, Pharmaceutical companies "Detail Reps" will give a number of "free samples" to the Hospital, Healthcare

Facilities, or even Specialists, which must be captured and recorded into the inventory system with ability to track dispensing by lot numbers in event of a recall, or adverse reactions reported by staff or the patient(s).

The point one should always remember is to make sure all documents are properly collected with necessary signatures from authorized individuals involved in the approval, ordering, delivery receipt, and inventory management. Careful handling of any documents required for completion of the "order to payment" cycle terms are critical because there is a high probability the Auditors will select one or more of those documents for review, but more importantly, it is protecting the assets of the organization.

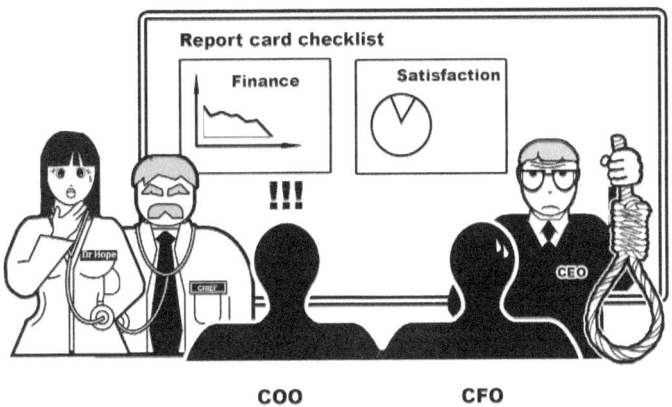

After this Audit is completed, we will give the Board a Report Card on the performance of the Management Team.
Good report card means continued employment;
Poor report card means "the noose".

13	Auditors and Audits should be perceived in a positive manner, as **they provide an independent, objective assessment of the financial and/or operational environment** and are able to identify "areas for improvement". They can be your "Report Card" of your performance.

We must appreciate the work of Auditors as they help ensure the organization is being managed properly, and they provide objective feedback of performance while asking probing questions about decisions taken (although this can be frustrating as they have the benefit of hindsight versus decisions that need to be taken with less than complete information) for issues that perhaps could have been managed better. However, the challenges cause everyone to review the circumstances and perhaps become learning points should a similar issue present in the future. In most instances, with proper explanations, most audit points under discussion will be resolved, and treated as minor; however, for those that are material, the Auditors will report them as part of the Management Letter to the Board for awareness and to be treated as areas for improvement, with action as required. Typically, Internal Audit Reports can be more revealing than external Management Letter and Points as Internal Auditors can spend more time investigating and testing, delving into details, both financial and operational. So, many more issues will be included in an Internal Audit Finding Report, and assigned priority numbers according to potential impact, and all points must be addressed by Senior Management to the satisfaction of the Board. External Audits are required to be performed to normally satisfy statutory and regulatory financial reporting requirements, e.g., Research and Operational Grants, Insurance, Company Registration, Charity, and Stock Exchange, etc. performing various standardized tests and sampling to give stockholders, stakeholders, and Board Members "comfort" that the Financial Statement fairly represents the position of the Organization or Company.

Results of both Internal and External Audit Reports provide the Boards (Directors or Trustees) with an objective assessment on the operational and financial performance of the Senior Management Team. Results are often taken into consideration as a key component in the annual appraisal of key Senior Management staff, and can affect their related emoluments (e.g. cash bonuses, stock options), entitlements (e.g., vehicles, transport, conferences etc.), and most important, employment contract renewals.

14 Remember for every audit performed, the Auditor's must report items and areas for improvement, so accept the fact. They have to justify their assignment and investment of resources to satisfy the defined audit scope. Knowing that, **minor Audit Point recommendations are welcomed. It is the major Audit Point shortfalls that need to be avoided**, and will cause discomfort and embarrassment to Senior Management and the Board.

Whenever there is either a operational (normally an Internal Audit) or financial audit (normally an External Audit) performed, the Auditors will generate a list of practices, procedures, entries, payments, documentation, internal controls, security lapses that may deviate from approved policies, procedures, or guidelines. Any identified non-compliance point provides an opportunity for someone (internal or external) to exploit the shortfall potentially culminating in a financial loss, breach of confidentiality, or damaging the reputation of the organization, or individuals.

There are so many activities, and transactions taking place in an organization, it is actually quite simple for an Auditor to find areas of non-compliance. This situation will occur even in the best run organizations, so there will be Audit Points identified. The important "screen" that each point must pass is to consider both materiality and potential impact to the organization should the point identified fail to be rectified. Therefore after an investment of time, and other resources as defined by the scope of the audit, there will be non-compliance findings. The outcomes will result in identification of weaknesses (areas for improvement) in the systems or procedures, and at time even certain "best practices" will be observed and commented upon. Most weaknesses will be classified on a five by five risk matrix, positioning each audit point on scale of one to five with the **impact** (materiality/magnitude) on the "x" axis, and the **likelihood** (probability) of occurrence on the "y" axis, with five on either axis being the most serious. All findings will be reported to Senior Management for clarification and determination if there are compensating measures in place to mitigate any potential negative outcomes which would justify not reporting the Audit Point. However, for all Audit points without sufficient mitigation features in place, they will be reported to Board for awareness. All Audit Points in the upper right quadrant of the matrix will require Management to develop immediate plans and a timetable to eliminate/avoid, reduce/ mitigate, or transfer the risk associated with the Audit Point.

Being in a C- Suit position (CEO, COO, CFO, CMB, CIO, CNO), they will work diligently to ensure any high level Audit Point is addressed and rectified as soon as possible and KIV (Keep In View) any lower valued Audit Point feedback and initiate action if any disturbing trends emerge.

So to close this section, any Audit will result in a certain number of Audit Points, of which they will be reported as either resolved or placed on a matrix to highlight the severity score. Any Audit that produces a "zero" non-compliance report would in itself be suspicious, so there will always be certain Audit Points highlighted for consideration and potential improvement. One cautionary note to share - any high level audit point reported and highlighted again in a subsequent year, is a major embarrassment to Senior Management charged with rectification from the prior year, and will usually have consequences. There must be documented plans and noticeable movement in addressing the issue(s).

15. Whenever a practicing Medical staff forms part of the Organization's Senior Clinical Leadership (CEO, CMB, Medical Director) **there must always be a balance between the specialty disciplines**, i.e., staff from the medical specialty and the staff from the surgical specialty side. They need to communicate, work together, and agree on actions to be taken. This helps to avoid perceived clinical bias in decisions taken by the general Clinical Staff of both Medical and Surgical disciplines. This is particularly important to avoid a perceived bias in Program development decisions.

In hospitals and healthcare facilities where both the CEO/MD and Chairman/Director of Medical Board are **practicing** Specialists, it helps to put in place a mechanism for the positions to be filled by a member of the opposite medical discipline, i.e. medical or surgical. This is especially true when the positions are filled by individuals who have been promoted through the ranks in the facility, or accepted appointments for the duties. This type situation occurs in both public and private hospital setting, and the issue is usually one of perception by the ranks of doctors under each discipline, rather than an actual, intentional bias by incumbents in the positions. This approach helps minimize the perception, and this only occurs when one or both individuals are practicing. If the Specialists have given up their active clinical practices, or are doctors who have previously chosen to take on administrative roles, then this situation usually does not appear to arise, nor the need for compensating actions to mitigate any negative or biased perceptions. Further, in most instances the CFO/FC will usually also work with a Group when discussing and evaluating CAPEX, and OPEX submissions, to ensure there is alignment with planned growth or new programs being introduced so there is also external support to help keep the balance, and focused on the objectives.

16   Whenever you are required to make presentations at Board Meetings, make sure time is taken to **brief key Members of the Board, e.g., Chairman, or Heads of various Sub-Committees on all the papers ahead of the meeting** to allow them to obtain an understanding of the issues to raised, and obtain their input before the Papers are finalized and distributed.

In preparation of making any presentations to the Board of Directors/Trustees for information/discussion/decision, one or more of Senior Management individuals attending the Board Meeting, individually or collectively should make an appointment to meet up with the Chairman of the Board/Trust to share a copy of the Paper/Presentation "deck of slides", and hold a discussion, particularly if any parts of the subject matter may be contentious or require background and understanding before taking a decision. Giving the Chairman an opportunity to be privately briefed allows him/her to ask questions, raise points for clarification, or add additional information if necessary. Involving them before the Board Meeting also allows them to suggest possible alternatives, or presentation approaches to make the Paper more presentable and acceptable to the other Board Members. The last thing you want is for your Chairman to be surprised by the proposals, and start questioning items, it is both distractive and destructive. If managed properly, Chairman should have a good understanding of the situation, proposed actions, and can even be in a position to provide support for the Paper, if it requires a decision, or may even answer questions from other Board Members, if they have not had sufficient time to understand the material.

Ensuring Chairman or other key Board Members have been personally briefed on Papers which could affect them or where their support is required, is a wise strategy. This briefing by Senior Management will avoid embarrassing situations where the Paper, Assumptions, Graphs and proposed outcomes are deliberated and "dissected" by either Board Chairman or key Chairmen of Board sub-Committees (e.g., Audit Committee, Remuneration, Manpower, Finance, Nomination, etc.). Better to provide a short presentation focusing on the salient points and ask Board Members for any comments. Normally, if the various Chairmen are knowledgeable of the information being presented, most other Members will defer to the most knowledgeable Members of the Board.

So always do your "lobbying" homework before any Board Meeting, by meeting with key Members who can influence the outcome of your Papers by informing, educating, and resolving any issues before hand. The best case is to ensure acceptance of the information or a desired decision. The worst case is to learn the Paper or proposal needs additional work before presenting.

17   Be serious when asked to serve as a **Mentor,** as it is both a great privilege and an opportunity to help **mold members of the next generation**, as well as recognition of your skills and contributions.

It is a privilege to be asked to be a Mentor in an official capacity. It should be recognized as a great honor and responsibility to be selected to train, coach, develop and mold future generations of upcoming professionals. Mentorship roles can be for a specific time period, or develop into long term relations lasting many years. Most medical staff often spend part or a sizeable amount of time in their professional careers in this type relationship (transfer of technology/knowledge skills), and are comfortable with the concept, while more senior administrative/management staff need to be exposed to the concept. Mentors should appreciate their role and responsibility in nurturing and cultivating the next generation in an actual working environment involving interactions about healthcare strategy, management techniques, operation optimization, financial assumptions, budgeting and accounting, as well as, IT and legal aspects relating to the organization. Senior Administrators must ultimately obtain exposure to, and understanding of all those areas. Formal educational knowledge acquired by staff either before or after joining the organization, still needs to be translated, interpreted, introduced, applied, tested, and measured to identify those that make a difference and move the organization ahead. Mentors play a key role in that processes and an appointment to provide that service and support should be welcomed by the individual(s) selected as recognition of their maturity and acquired skills, so should not be viewed as "just another duty". Mentors should also be individuals who can provide personal, one-on-one counseling to their charges, helping them understand their capabilities, think through and resolve conflicts, and providing direction in developing their potential based on their personal career aspirations. These aspirations can range from wanting to achieve and succeed to more senior levels within the organization/ industry, or simply develop their skills to be the "best they can be" in their current level, and support the Senior Administrators. Individuals/ Mentees can choose roles to best contribute to the organization and support their senior staff in achieving organizational goals, while maintaining their personal work-life balance targets, without having "political or other conflicting aspirational agendas" that work against their bosses. This is a great comfort for the boss to know their key support/reporting staff (next line down) are complementing their efforts and not competing with them.

It is a privilege to have several Mentors over the course of one's professional development and growth, offering guidance in specific/specialized areas such as clinical, nursing, or other professional and administrative areas. Over the years Mentor relationships should have provided guidance to help develop their charges to assume new and expanded roles, and become the successors to existing senior management within professional departments of the organization, or given an opportunity to apply their skills at another or new facility.

A Mentor's greatest legacy is to be "remembered" as an individual who helped develop, influence and instill the correct principles in the next generation of staff.

18 Be alert - The time when **most crisis occur** (in the hospital/clinic/admin) is **within the last two hours before start of the weekend**, Public Holiday, or whenever you plan to go on Annual Leave.

It is common for issues to be raised or a crisis to be elevated to Senior Management over a perceived or actual medical management or treatment issue, as well as other administrative management shortfalls towards the end of week. Ironically, this periodically occurs just before you are planning to be away, and requires your urgent attention. Once this occurs, one must be prepared to take the necessary decisions, and actions to either close the issue or develop alternate solutions. Obviously, the most serious situations may require one to delay, reschedule, or cancel the plans. The information source of the "crisis" can arise from either internal or external parties, specifically, individual staff within the organization, or through external parties, such as the Board, Media, or Government Body such as Ministry/Department of Health or equivalent.

"Why do these issues occur at the most inopportune times, the last minute?", is a question often asked; and the best explanation appears to be that junior staff level individuals (anything below Senior Management) have attempted but were unable to resolve the issue(s) or reached an impasse, so the matter is "escalated" to higher levels for timely solution; hence, landing on your desk just before the weekend, or just before you are planning to go on leave.

Over the years, many solutions have been implemented to minimize the risk of this occurring on a regular basis, and at the last minute.

18.1 Have a robust "incident reporting system" in place that captures any incident within hours or even minutes of occurrence. This provides an "early warning" system as well as an opportunity to start the resolution process, avoiding last minute surprises,

18.2 Promote a culture of communication, by having responsible staff raise issue(s) to their respective Manager, who then assesses the situation and provides a verbal update to Senior Management, both to alert them and obtain guidance as necessary minimizing, the surprise element and impact,

18.3 Make sure there is a clear structure within the Departments and Organization where alternative staff (Number Twos) can be developed over time to assume responsibility for addressing the issue, and taking the necessary decisions and actions to resolve or escalate the matter,

18.4 Implement a culture of "empowerment" where staff are given authority to make decisions such as adjustments, and waivers, at amounts appropriate with their position and the "value of the issue" being contested,

18.5 Ensure staff are reminded to be alert and vigilant for the entire time they are at work,

18.6 Develop a "network" of individuals, and counterparts in other Healthcare Facilities and, Ministries who may become aware of emerging issues before they are "formally" brought to your attention,

18.7 Encourage and make efforts for Corporate Communications to develop contacts and relationships with the Media segment, so Reporters and Journalists will make contact to seek or clarify information, and perhaps avert, mitigate, or resolve issues with proper information and being brought up in the news. Certain Senior Management staff should also be involved in this relationship building.

So, with a good infrastructure and planning most clinical and management crisis situations can be managed.

19 Make sure your supporters are **AHEAD** of you or **WITH** you. Be wary of supporters who are always **100% BEHIND** you as you do not know how far behind they are, what is in their hand, or what they are saying.

This is a variant of an old saying, but putting perspective on where your supporters are positioned. Unfortunately, in the real world, while individuals will claim support of your position, idea, recommendation, it is better if they are visibly alongside you, as there are times when other individuals will present "logical" arguments that may cause your Supporters to the change their position, and when it comes to "crunch time" you learn that the Supporter has changed position. This unknown change is referred to as "stabbing you in the back". One should keep your Supporters constantly updated on the sequence of any events (good and bad) where you need their commitment, providing proper explanations to obtain a sense of any change in attitude or position regarding their support and actively seek their feedback on issues/questions being raised "on the ground". Better to know ahead of time, and perform "damage control" or at worst, know the type of opposition or questions that will be raised to potentially derail your initiative and potentially embarrass you whether at a presentations to the Board, Staff or public.

20   Too much effort is spent **CHASING** others to get things done, when what we really need is to **CATCH** them (individuals involved).

It is a common expression staff often use when questioned about the status of an "open item" being discussed, e.g., status of a long outstanding patient bill payment, delay in receipt of grant funding, delay in organization making timely payments, receipt of overdue goods and equipment to close outstanding Purchase Orders, delay/failure in developing a process, procedure, or implementing a clinical or operational program, etc. The staff would reply they would "chase" the relevant parties to achieve the objectives. My response to their comment is the word "chase" connotes an action that means we are behind, and unable to close the gap. So I correct staff to say we want to "catch" (identify) the individuals involved and agree on expected actions to be taken to achieve closure.

So a better term would be to "follow-up" with the relevant parties within a specific time (one day/week/month) period to give it a sense of urgency, and take the necessary action to resolve any obstacles and remove this as an open/outstanding item.

21 Notice that Taxies always **DRY UP** when it rains....

This is a more practical than profound observation regarding taxies, having had to depend on them for many years as a primary mode of transport. During dry, non-raining days taxies often queue at designated Taxi Stands, or are available on relatively short notice when you call. Suddenly when it rains, they tend to become unavailable "dry-up" both at Taxi Stands and for call in "bookings", resulting in long queue waits, and in many instances, being late for meetings. The obvious reason is that many commuters who regularly use others modes of transportation such as walking, buses, and MRT (Metro) decide to use taxies to minimize getting wet when traveling to other business locations, or returning home after work. The same observations apply to the Uber, Grab, and other similar transport services, so the point is just a reminder to make allowances in time to compensate for the expected delays and avoid getting "stressed out" when going to/from work or to meetings during the day.

22   **The computer, program, or printer always "hangs"**, or runs out of ink when you are in a hurry.

Here is another experience belonging to Murphy's Law compendium of "things that can go wrong, will". There are occasions when after a presentation, a document(s) must be prepared or modified and produced for signature by the close of a meeting to capture the results of the negotiation, or formal agreement discussion. In the rush to finalize the document "something" happens to the computer (e.g., battery goes "flat" and no power cable immediately available); the software program "freezes up" usually do to issues with version compatibility, alternatively, the printer runs out of ink or paper somewhere in the midst of printing multiple page documents, or it loses the "Wi-Fi" connection. All of which cause unnecessary delays and raises stress levels of the individuals trying to prepare the documents, while creating a palpable uneasiness amongst the individuals waiting to sign the documents.

The best way to minimize the above problems from occurring is to ensure one staff is tasked to visually check, and test the working condition of the equipment to be used before the meeting, as well as, a stock of required supplies. A thorough inspection should pick up any obvious potential shortcoming. Another option periodically used is to have additional equipment made available as a back-up, having the same configurations and can be activated on short notice.

With regards to software compatibility, at least one or two computers in the organization should be of the latest high end model and configured with the latest software and hardware versions available. This is especially relevant when presentation and programs involving international participants, Senior Organization Members, or other Officials. Certain organization (local and international), use the latest versions, and if hosting organization has yet to adopt the latest version, this may introduce a compatibility issue when running their software or data programs. These high end computers are usually located in the Corporate Communications or Education & Training Departments since they normally "take the lead" in preparing for presentation activities.

23 Remember all **Administrators/Managers/Senior Managers** are really **Janitors**. Their role is to clean up messes and keep their areas clean, so they should never lose their perspective.

The role of all Administrators, Senior Managers, and Managers is to resolve problems and issues under their area or scope of responsibility. Their effectiveness and efficiency is often measured and rewarded based on their documented resolutions of outstanding problems or handling of situations that emerged during the year. In many instances new individuals are given the task to "clean up the mess" of a previous incumbent who for whatever reason allowed multiple conditions to arise, that they failed to resolve. Essentially all Managers and above are responsible to ensure their respective areas are kept in order, lines of communication are "kept open", and contribute to the success and performance of the organization. As a result, Managers and above, looking at their roles from a functional perspective are to keep the place clean and free of any operational obstructions and procedural "clutter" which is also the basic Job Description of Janitorial/Environmental staff, but having a different level of responsibility with a broader scope. Hence, we serve as organizational "Janitors"!

24 **Insurance coverage frequently lapses**, for whatever reason, shortly before you need to make a claim.

This is an interesting situation that has occurred both at work, and in a personal capacity. Any remedial action is dependent on the amount of time that the insurance coverage has lapsed. If the time period is short, periodically the insurance company has the flexibility to assist with several options, i.e., allow for making an interim payment to extend the previous policy, or issue a new renewal policy with an effective date immediately after the expiry of the previous policy. This must normally occur within 30 days from the expiry date of the policy. If your organization has had a long term coverage relationship, the insurance company will try to assist. Better still, the insurance company should send out reminders of policies nearing expiration if the renewal payments have yet to be received as the expiry date approaches. This type of situation cannot be a regular occurrence, so all internal processes must be refined to avoid a repeat. It is recommended the insurance expiry dates for all policies being managed by the organization be reviewed monthly and take decisions (cancel/lapse, renew) on any policies scheduled to expire within the next 90 days.

Unfortunately, if the expiration is too long, there may be no immediate insurance solution to the problem, so at the company level it may require making a full "out of pocket" payment for the cost that would normally have been covered by the insurance claim, after any deductible or co-payment is taken into consideration. If the outlay is not too large it may be amortized over the remaining months of the current financial year as part of normal operating costs. However, if the amount is material, it may require approval of the Board, to make the payment depending on the approval level hierarchy within the organization and the financial impact of the uncovered claim or replacement costs. This will require the necessary disclosure to the Board on the circumstances, and any corrective action taken, or to be taken.

25   Interesting observation to note, people who live closest to work or work closest to where a meeting is being held, **are typically the ones who are late** (or cannot make it in), for work or the meeting!

This is an interesting observation experienced at different locations I have worked on an international basis.

A hospital is a 24x7 day operation, and does not shut down for weather or other external activities. There are patients who are depending on medical, nursing and other therapeutic professionals, as well as, support staff who ensure patients are fed, rooms cleaned, linens changed, and other hospitality type activities are performed. Staff who accept work in the hospital must understand that fact when they start working, so they must be prepared to make a commitment. When one takes a position in a hospital, they should consider aspects such as distance, and have several alternative access routes identified to the hospital (to get to work).

When we lived In the "cold" countries where it snowed, sometimes heavily, it was often the individuals who lived closest to the hospital who would call in to request to take the day off, citing the snow as the impediment in terms to making it to work, and requesting management to declare it a "snow day", so the time off would not be charged against their annual leave. Unfortunate for them when the requests came to me, I indicated if they wished to take the day off, they had to make arrangements for someone else to cover their duties and they would be required to submit a request for annual leave to cover the day(s) off. With those two conditions, most made it into work, albeit a bit late. The reason for the position taken is that I lived about 10 miles (16 kms) from the office, and if I could make it in, I expected the other staff could do the same when they lived much closer. One just needed to make allowance for the additional time required, i.e. arise earlier, leave earlier for work, etc. If there was a real emergency, such as a blizzard, deep snow, flood, storm, hurricane, tornado, etc. the local and regional governmental authorities would declare a "weather emergency" and issue advisories for people to limit travel or remain home. In those rare instances, all staff in the hospital would be required to continue working, arranging time to get some sleep in the hospital, where food was provided. Other than under those conditions, hospital staff are expected to report and assume their duties. So consideration for weather related excuses must be carefully evaluated, to the detriment of staff currently in the hospital.

The other more prevalent and more relevant situation is when a meeting is being held at your facility and the meeting location is within in the same building, or in relatively close proximity of the Head/Chairperson of the Meeting. Individuals attending the meeting from other facilities will tend to take into consideration travel time, i.e. leaving their offices in sufficient time, and almost always be on time or early for the meeting. However, staff within the hosting facility often believe since they are so close, they can continue to work until everyone is assembled and about ready to start the meeting. Rather than being early to greet everyone, and make sure everything is in working order, what generally happens is that they continue to work, forgetting the time, or a taking a telephone call, or talking with an individual who walks into their office with a question or issue that requires time to resolve, rather than defer that discussion or delegate it to another staff. As a result, instead of starting the meeting on time, all the others participants must wait for the Chairman/Head or key member of the Workgroup before starting, which is expensive (cumulative value of remuneration of all participants) and makes the others who traveled from a distance spend more time away from their respective offices than necessary.

The point is, everyone's time is precious, and further, we must be sensitive and professional to the needs of the Meeting Attendees, so local staff leading the Meeting must always be mindful of their commitment to ensure all services are available and provided to the best of the organization's ability. It is also an image situation.

26 It is better to be remembered as being a Great **Number Two**, than as a Poor or Mediocre **Number One.**

Many individuals have as part of their career plan, the objective of securing the number one position of the "C Suite", positions, specifically CEO or MD, CMB, COO, CFO, CNO, CIO or their equivalents in an organization, which is good for both parties, as it keeps the individuals motivated, and for the organization, it offers potential succession planning and replenishment of talent. The rise to the most senior positions also requires assuming of more and more responsibility, including holistic understanding of the organization, visionary strategic planning, and comfort in facing and managing the Board, Stockholders, Stakeholders, public and media. Individuals in those roles must have the necessary personality to be the "face" of the organization and comfortable with commitments for presentations to both the Board and external organizations, attending functions on almost a daily basis, long hours, traveling, arbitrating/negotiation with various groups, recruitment of key reporting staff, living with difficult decisions to downsize the organization or terminate/release individuals which impacts many lives and livelihoods, as well as managing different "political" situations either within the organization or external. Successful fulfillment of those expectations will define their legacy and contribution once they step down.

There are many individuals who have successfully achieved their career aspiration of attaining the "C Suite" position, only to learn they are unable to meet all the defined expectations, and become tired or frustrated, and must deal with the realization of the "toll" it can take on them personally and/or their family life. If they can honestly recognize their incompatibility in the role, they can let it be known they wish to take on a different supportive role, such as one of the positions reporting directly to the CEO/MD, CMB, COO, CFO, CNO, CIO and can then focus their attention, skills, and strengths to support them, and can even provide temporary or interim coverage, and be remembered as a great "Number Two" person who supported and help make the Number One position perform better. The alternative is to resign, often stated in euphuistic phrase "resigning to pursue other interests".

This realization is aligned with an old concept called the "Peter Principle[1]" which stated, "In a hierarchy Every Employee Tends to Rise to His Level of Incompetence". That means, good employees tend to be promoted and rise to the point or level they become ineffective in performing their duties. Unfortunately, many promotions are based on past performance, time in grade/service and/or in a capacity not directly related to the abilities required for the position (e.g. good/excellent Clinician or Nurse does not automatically equate to be a good Administrator) for which they are being promoted within the same or different industry. Once one moves into positions or levels for which they cannot manage or cope, they will become unproductive and a "stumbling block" for the organization to progress further. This is very serious for those in the most senior positions. So, if you find yourself in this situation, it is better to find and fill a supporting position that can benefit from your best qualities and allows you to become a treasured staff within the organization. As an added benefit, the Number One is not threatened by you, and a great working and supportive relationship can be developed to benefit both.

27   The clever Leader **capitalizes** on a subordinate's **strengths**, and **complements any weaknesses** by either developing the individual, or hiring staff with the necessary skills to form a Team.

---

1   "The Peter Principle", Laurence J. Peter, Raymond Hull, 1969

One of the characteristics of an astute Leader, CEO level or equivalent within the organization, is the fact they know they have limitations in their skillsets or gaps in their management coverage, so they make efforts to recruit individuals who complement their weaknesses, ultimately building a powerful Team who can address and manage most situations. With that basic approach, the Leader has comfort the individuals are professional, thereby allowing the Leader to focus on the strategic directions for the organization and meeting the Board's expectation.

In the recruitment process, the Manager must make a special effort to identify and select individuals who display both the necessary basic and advanced skillsets who can be further nurtured and developed so they at some point be qualified to replace them (concept of training your replacement to allow oneself to be promoted). To achieve this objective, at times it means taking initiative to engage one or more professional "headhunter" Firms to assist in that search for the best individual. In the long term, it is a very satisfying feeling and a complement to the Leader when one of their key staff is selected for a more senior position within the current organization or another one as the Leader has expanded and contributed to the total number of Senior professionals in the healthcare industry!

The message here is for the Leader to build a solid cohesive, integrated Team, whose members skills complement each other and move the organization to new levels.

28   **Loyalty** and commitment from staff **should be recognized** and appreciated.

Staff who faithfully support their supervisors, managers, and organizational initiatives and directions are valuable, as they will make the necessary contribution in time and effort to ensure the company remains viable. Loyalty can be demonstrated by the junior staff who perform their work to the "highest standards" and help ensure the customer/patient achieve the best experience in their journey through the healthcare system. Similar support will be given by the mid and upper levels of staff, working toward the performance objectives. For senior managers and key organization individuals, it is their efforts in strategically planning for the company's future based on the expressed directions of the Board/Trustees and ensuring the necessary efforts are being taken. Many staff do this "out of loyalty and commitment" to the organization and their personal desire to participate in its achievements and pride in its success. On that basis, senior management of the organization should periodically take time to recognize the efforts of staff in that process. Recognition of their loyalty, can take many forms, both in non-monetary as well as monetary ways.

Non-monetary recognition can be a simple as Senior Management walking the grounds, observing work staff are performing and proving instant feedback on their good work. It can also be by publishing staff names and specials efforts taken in internal newsletters and updates. More structured avenues of loyalty recognition and contribution can be in nominating staff for Organization and/or Group recognition, where invitations to dinners or other outings specifically targeting the loyal staff in the organization.

Monetary recognition can come through via the annual appraisal process, with a portion of their bonus being a function of the individual's demonstrated commitment, faithfulness, and dedication to the organization. Annual Awards ceremonies where recognition is given along with monetary "tokens" of appreciation are also a common methodology to promote awareness. All these efforts bring recognition to the loyal staff, their subordinates, and peers by being role models, as well as a source of pride to their supervisors. Loyalty recognition must also include the organization's Partners and their staff, as without their loyalty and commitment, their service will not be appreciated.

The takeaway point is to remind supervisors, managers, and senior staff to take time to observe and appreciate staff and write up or nominate individuals and give it to the Human Resources Department to collate, and help develop models to recognize staff, organize activities to "spread the word" of the loyalty and commitment, both within the Organization, Corporate Group, Professional Societies, and Industry.

29   Whenever asked about availability, "I am **never free, but affordable**".

Time of all individuals is a valuable commodity; however, depending on the issue or questions to be asked, and the estimated amount of time required for a short meeting or discussion, I would always tell my staff that I am never free, but affordable in term of access and willingness to work or help them with a question or problem. Being free connotes that I am sitting around with nothing to do, just waiting for their call. I would always make attempts to meet up with my staff, or anyone else with a reasonable request, to assist, but it may not be immediate but within a reasonable time. As a Senior Member of the organization, we should never forget the time value of providing services or guidance, but at the same time one should make time to meet with superiors, peers, .direct reports, and subordinates to facilitate communications and problem solving.

30 Observation. During a Conference/Seminar, always ensure there is an individual **who can manage the various audio-visual components** available, as the moment they are not around, something will go wrong! Thanks to Murphy!

At some point during a conference, seminar, or important internal presentation, a problem with the audio-visual, or computer program will arise and may cause some delay or disruption in the continuity of the presentation. While it is critical to have all the systems checked before the beginning of the program, it is also important to check the operational performance before each new speaker begins their topic presentation. Make sure the "thumb drive or other storage media" file opens properly, if only inserted immediately before the presentation or for pre-installed files, ensure it is accessible, loads properly, and working. Take the responsibility to personally ensure there are necessary individuals in attendance, or on standby immediately outside the presentation venue (if the presentation is confidential) who have the necessary technical skills to address any situation that may arise, and when they do, minimize any disruption in the program delivery. If not proactively managed, this is one situation that will qualify as a "Murphy's Law" experience. Further, the probability for this type of situation to occur will increase if any speakers or presenters are from different countries where they may be using a different version of the same software (most likely a newer version) which may be incompatible with the software version or local equipment hardware configuration at the conference, seminar, or presentation location. This can be very frustrating. The proactive way to manage this type situation is to ensure at least one computer in the organization, or presentation site (conference, seminar, auditorium, Board Room, etc.) is configured to accommodate the latest version of any software commonly used, as the newest and most advanced software is normally compatible with lower versions. This approach may require periodically upgrading or investing in new computer systems with latest hardware configuration, as many new software versions require more space to accommodate the program. So, forward planning and investment, along with skilled staff being nearby, will minimize the potential of any problem occurring, and keep Murphy from raising his head, while ensuring successful presentations!

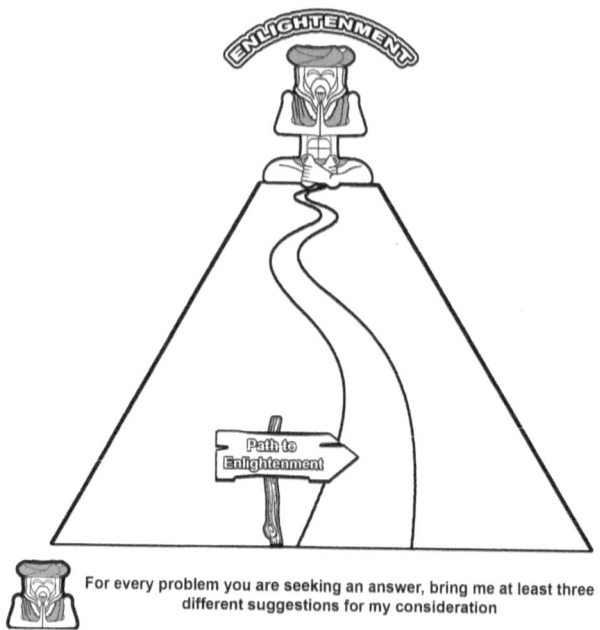

For every problem you are seeking an answer, bring me at least three different suggestions for my consideration

31 Inculcate into your reporting staff the following concept/practice - **"Bring me a problem, bring me at least three workable/operational solutions"** for consideration. This way, staff become invested by thinking about the situation and can often facilitate in the solution as they are closest to the problem. The final solution you approve may be a validation of what was proposed, a variant, or a combination.

Early in my career I learned from my supervisor/mentor that for every issue or problem I raised, a solution was within my sphere of control or responsibility, so I should always think about potential solutions. Over the years I adopted a mantra of "bring me a problem, bring me at least three potential, workable solutions" as a good approach to train my staff. I required them to think of potential solutions based on their perspectives of the situation, both within and "outside the box". This process also developed the staff to think critically, and not merely pass the problem to another level, either up or down. Often as a direct supervisor, or higher, it is difficult to relate to specific problems at the ground level, so input from staff at that level is both rewarding and helpful. This concept can be applied all the way through the organization from the ground level staff to senior management. I found when one of their solution proposals (part or all) is implemented; staff take more pride and ownership to make it work. I also personally adopted the same principle when making proposals to my superiors in Senior Management or even the Board, often time even more than three (as many as six to ten) to provide a comprehensive perspective.

When crafting the three solutions, they must be realistic, and workable. A "do nothing" solution is a solution, but becomes number four or five or "x" and does not normally qualify to satisfy the one of three solutions requirement objective, even though it may be taken into consideration. What I am always looking for, is a solution that addresses the core or root problem, and what are the positive (pro) merits and negative (con) implications of each solution proposed. Once the issues and resultant solutions are presented and discussed, there are various potential outcomes, ranging from adopting one of the solutions in its entirety as proposed, modified with elements of other solutions, or adopting a "best practice" within or outside the industry, as well as consideration of the current situation. Even the basic three solutions required can be increased by merging several singular solutions, resulting with more variants for consideration. From a Senior Manager level perspective, I am looking for the individuals or team who takes this advice seriously and come up with workable creative and innovative outcomes.

Within many organizations, over the past 15-20 years there have been initiatives to encourage similar thought, analysis and solutions. Often, Teams are formed to compete in addressing different problems and developing the best solutions. All successful outcomes make the Team Members winners, as well as the organization, and ultimately our patients who benefit from any improvements.

> 32   Recommendation. When managing professional level subordinates, it is best to **adopt an "eclectic style" of Management**, built on each staff's strengths, and know what "buttons to push" to obtain their best performance.

Effectively, in a hospital or healthcare setting, all staff have specific tasks and roles to perform, and they need to be responsive to the ever changing needs of patients and operational conditions. So as Managers, Senior Managers and above, we must recruit and work toward developing our direct reports to perform at their roles to the best of their abilities. As Management, we need to learn each individual's strong and weak characteristics and provide direction that is tailored to their learning styles. Certain individuals learn and respond better with visual aids, or auditory presentations. Others learn better through action methods such as writing/note taking, and "hands on" projects. While all professional level subordinate should have exposure to and use various techniques to carry out their respective responsibilities, it is our responsibility to 'know our staff" and which methods they respond to best. So, that means we must vary our approaches in managing each of them to capitalize on their respective strengths and help them develop in areas of their weaknesses. This is called an eclectic style of management, in contrast to using an "assembly line" or "cookie cutter" approach when managing our staff. This is particularly important with professional level staff development as the objective is to encourage staff to learn different approaches and think creatively to address issues. The "assembly line" approach works fine when introducing a new basic approach or technology, such as learning a new software program, or assembly technique, but is of little or no value when encouraging direct reports to take initiative to complete projects or assignments. I want to point them in the correct direction, but avoid doing the work for them, but I will invest time using techniques that facilitate in their grasping necessary concepts and ideas.

Therefore remember, find the "buttons" you need to press to encourage and develop your direct reports, to make them better managers, and be more productive.

33 Responsibility of **taking Minutes (Notes) of Meetings is under appreciated**. While the Minute Taker must ensure both accuracy and completeness in substance and spirit, judicious use of words and sentence structure provides ability to influence the tone and responsibility. Be happy to take Minutes (Notes)!

In many organizations the task of recording Minutes or Notes of Meetings is often delegated to the Secretaries or Executives. If it is your Secretary or Personal Assistant (PA), it normally is not an issue, but if an Executive or any other individual takes the Minutes or Notes you must be sure to read and edit them carefully. At times you may be meeting with more senior staff or participating in a very confidential meeting discussing sensitive matters, you may be requested to take the Minutes or Notes. If not asked, offer to take the Minutes or Notes.

Either taking or vetting of Minutes or Notes gives one the ability to capture items and present the key points in the best manner and interpretation possible. At times Minutes can be used as proof should any future disagreement arise, so responsibility for accuracy is crucial. Should individuals who are outside of your direct supervision or responsibility take the Minutes or Notes, make sure you have the opportunity to "review" them while in draft mode, before being circulated and finalized to ensure they are complete and accurate. Once finalized, all participants will be bound to the information recorded. While not intentional, even one word misplaced or misused can change the meaning, context, or content to which you will be bound, so take the responsibility seriously.

34   A **Successor must always make changes**, to demonstrate they are making a difference.

Whenever there is a change in Senior Management (CEO/MD, CFO, COO, CMB, CNO, CIO, or equivalents) there will inevitably be changes in policies and expectations. Change in Senior Management is usually due to strategic

Board rotational expectations, as well as good governance to ensure the organization is periodically re-energized and refreshed. Most often the new Management Team or selected individuals may have relevant proven experience, and may even be relatively younger than the outgoing Team, or Individual. In all instances, the Board or Senior Management will give instructions to achieve specific improvements or changes as part of their appointment brief in areas such as, strategic directions, clinical quality, clinical performance/outcomes, resolving outstanding financial situations, manpower related issues, achieving workload or performance optimization, improving operational efficiencies, introducing new programs, and expanding market share, etc. So by virtue of the new Individual or Team's expectations, management changes will occur so the newly appointed Individuals will be able to meet their expected objective(s) which translates into continued engagement in their respective roles. As no organization is perfect, there will always be areas for improvement and change, so subsequent changes should not be taken personally. One must also expect that there will be "perception and personality differences" that will ultimately result in certain incumbent staff leaving the organization.

35   The best way to **learn the effectiveness of signage within and around the hospital** or healthcare facility is to task new recruits with assignments that require them to navigate throughout the facility during their first couple weeks, and provide feedback on their experiences, then "fill in the gaps".

This is a simple but useful exercise to evaluate the effectiveness of your signage within and around the hospital or medical facility. Often, when patients, visitors, vendors, or general public move around a facility, particularly for the first time, they frequently become frustrated in trying to arrive at a particular location, such as a ward, clinic, or service department (Imaging, Pharmacy, Rehabilitation) and end up asking for directions. Some individuals will give feedback, while others will just grumble to their friends or relatives on the difficulties experienced.

So, as part of the "New Staff Orientation", individuals will be required to participate in several "games" where each is given a different list of five locations they need to "find", and must complete the assignment within 10 to15 minutes. Each staff starts at one of the entrances to the facility, and records their progress using only available signage, without asking for any assistance. Upon completion, a debrief is held where staff share their "feedback" both positive and negative which are passed to Facilities Management to review and improve signage and eliminate "blind spots", or visibility issues.

Signage protocol requires signs to be within "line of sight" of the next sign, new so staff serve as proxies for patients trying to move around the facility. If staff can locate their destination without issue, then the signage is most likely good; however, if there is any difficulty encountered, then the signage (visibility, adequacy, size, color, font size, contrast, gaps, positioning, frequency, use of pictograms, etc.) must be revised. Over time, and with regular feedback from the new staff, patterns will be identified, so the signage can be improved.

It is important to use new staff within the first few days or week after joining, because any longer, staff will become familiar with routes and shortcuts to many locations, so they lose objectivity, perspective, and challenges faced by first time patients and others.

Contribute by making suggestion to improve the navigation journey through the hospital or healthcare facility convenient as possible for the patient or accompanying caregiver.

36   Ensure all subordinate staff understand the necessity of keeping their immediate superior updated and appraised of any potential condition or situation that may arise that could be brought to your Supervisor's attention. **Your Supervisor should never learn of an important or emerging issue in your area of responsibility from a Superior or Outsider before you are aware of the situation. This is called being "blind-sided"**, and reflects poorly on you and your staff's communication.

It is a most embarrassing situation when you are called into your boss's office, or queried by a Board Member on an emerging issue brought to their attention, that you have not heard anything about, and cannot intelligently answer! Indicating you will investigate and revert back is an interim answer, but actually reflects poorly on you and your control of the chain of command as there has been a breakdown in communication flow. Every individual in a supervisory position in the organization's reporting hierarchy must keep their respective supervisor's informed of any condition where there is the potential of causing harm or creating an embarrassment should it become knowledge to any external party, who then queries individuals of the organization, from the Board on down. Failure of being kept informed of relevant operational pieces of information, both good and bad, by your subordinates results in you or your boss being "blindsided" (i.e., not being aware of a situation when asked). Worse still is the situation where you were aware of a situation and failed to update your boss or superior. As responsible management and supervisory individuals, it is our duty to share information with relevant individuals in the organization both to protect ourselves, our bosses, and the organization as the sharing of relevant information will generate discussion on how to manage the situation. If the information is positive, then plans should be drawn up to share the information with other Members of the Board, and then plan for Press Releases to the media at an appropriate time. For negative information situations, proactive actions should be started immediately to address the situation, so when briefing more senior individuals in the Board (or Ministry) they are made aware of the mitigating efforts being taken, so when questioned about the situation, an intelligent reply can be offered. I would always tell my staff, that the worst thing they can do to me is allow me to be "blindsided" of an issue they were aware of, and failed to bring to my attention. Staff in Managerial positions should have sufficient experience and maturity to discern when an issue or information should be shared. Depending on the situation, the information can be shared at the next "internal meeting or update" but if the situation is of a serious nature, the information must be shared immediately, regardless of the time (even if in the middle of the night) and wherever you may be (at home, holiday, conference).

Necessary meetings both internal and external can then be initiated to strategize and formulate what actions to take.

Remember, you have the responsibility to ensure your boss is apprised of any significant or meaningful event or situation that comes to your attention, keeping them from being blindsided, and leave the "plausible deniability" defense to the military and government sectors. It is better to be "over-briefed" of a situation from one or more staff, as then we know we are communicating and calibrating, so we can take the necessary decision about notification of the appropriate individuals.

37 It is easier to **"sell a concept or idea"** and instill a sense of ownership, when all parties are **given an opportunity to "flesh out" an idea**.

New concepts and ideas to improve the organization or treating patients are always occurring. The concepts and ideas may come from both internal and external sources. When a decision is taken to adopt them, it is necessary to present and engage all staff who are required to support them. This is not always an easy tasks as the new concepts and tasks may confront established concepts and practices and result in tension and resistance. To make a successful transition, it requires and understanding of the new concepts and ideas. A proven and successful tactic used by consultants, educators, and management is to engage all the key individuals who will be tasked with managing and implementing the new concepts and obtain their input do develop the process, and identify outcome metrics to be achieved. When they are involved in that process several things happen. First, the participants obtain a better understanding of the new concept or idea, and have an opportunity to question, challenge, and participate in resolving the necessary issues by providing input to "flesh out" the process. Once completed, this should lead to a "sense of ownership" because they can recognize their contributions and were involved. This approach works with professionals, and management, as well as line staff within departments to ensure a 360° perspective is achieved. By engaging the staff, it may require an investment in time up front, but will ultimately be implemented with less resistance and time spent revising and modifying. By the way, everything is dynamic, so over time concepts and ideas must be re-evaluated and re-validated.

38   **Transparency builds** responsibility and accountability.

Transparency in operational and financial aspects generates an openness so the thought process can be understood, learn if the best solutions, and most efficient processes have been considered and applied. Transparency is also required when managing patients or clients, but the processes are different. In general, transparency is expected to create an atmosphere of openness and understanding.

From the operational financial perspective, business transparency results in sharing of key information, algorithms, assumption rationale to validate any approach taken and conclusions formed to ensure the best results are being achieved. With transparency, it is easier to isolate the key business "drivers" and who is in the position to influence the target outcomes, so they can be given responsibility to take necessary actions which can impact on the performance (and profits) of the organization. Internal operational and financial models should be designed to allow for "sensitivity analysis" where by adjusting various assumptions it is possible to assess the impact. Once the input is adjusted to achieve the best, realistic outcome, then tasks can be assigned and accountability given for achieving the performance target set. With this approach after a requisite time has elapsed, if an outcome different from what was expected/projected, it is easier to determine the cause of the variation, and whether it was within control, or an unplanned, external situation occurred created a deviation. With that information, it is much easier to explain while becoming a learning point for future analysis, as well as the performance evaluation of the individuals involved. This approach can be used at either Department or Organization level.

The opposite of the transparency mode is the "black hole" concept which is completely opaque, confusing and generates loss of support, understanding, and confidence. This approach is normally observed in an autocratic management environment, and fails to allow for discussion, denying new generations of professional being groomed an opportunity to learn. There is no mentoring or transfer of knowledge in this model and the creative staff will ultimately leave the organization in frustration, leaving only staff who want to be directed.

Achieving a transparent environment is also important when managing patients/clients for them to understand treatment options available, as the processes and charges to be incurred for each option as there may be a substantial treatment modalities and costs differences. This requires the clinical/medical, nursing, and other professional staff share information about the patient's treatment, care, and potential outcomes. At times, professional staff are of the opinion the patient, or caregiver(s) is not able to understand or process the information, whether clinical or financial in nature; however, it is critical to the patient and caregiver, so they can make informed decisions about their treatment options! Further, if managed correctly and openly, this will reduce misunderstandings and frustration when handling the patient and family, particularly if the outcome differs from the expected, and when they receive their bills for services provided as they were involved in the treatment decisions.

So the importance of the initial simple statement is to foster an environment of being open and transparent in all actions, analysis, and dealings should lead to better understanding and acceptance of outcomes throughout the organization.

39   What actions can Hospitals and Healthcare Facilities undertake to **Manage Expired and/or Returned Medications** from patients.

For many years management of returned and expired drugs for patients had been a difficult matter.

Most hospitals and healthcare facilities had strict "no return" policies, about acceptance once drugs and medications were issued, so this policy effectively closed off most patients from any return possibility, unless a drug was found to have a contra-indication notice about taking it with another medication prescribed to the same patient. Only in those infrequent instances were the drugs taken back and new, replacement drug issued.

Certain Doctor and Specialist practice patterns were observed whereby patients were allowed to collect the full quantity of drug prescribed at one time up to one year in advance, under the pretext of being more convenient by removing the need for the patient or caregivers to come back for periodic refills.

Frequently feedback was received from frustrated patients and families who offered many reasons for consideration to allow return or replacement of various quantities of drugs and medications, such as, too much to store, no longer effective, doctor or Specialists prescribed a new set of drugs and medications, or even the fact that the patient "passed away" and there was a substantial supply remaining.

As hospitals and healthcare facilities became more patient sensitive, hospitals started making exceptions and taking back various unused drugs giving partial or complete credit on a "goodwill" basis. However, the drugs and medications taken back were isolated and destroyed as they could never be reissued due to legal liability issues (since it was impossible to answer how they were kept, i.e., where they were stored, under what conditions), and serious concerns about potential tampering.

During review of the Pharmacy's inventory movement, it came to Management's attention these new practices were impacting by increasing cost, so Finance initiated a review of costs to quantify the financial impact of the new practice. Meetings were held with Senior Clinical Management and together they came up with a "pilot study" to issue only a limited quantity of medications and only for specified periods of time, e.g., from one week to a maximum of three to four months duration, but it did require periodic visits to the Pharmacy to obtain the next allotment, sometimes after a brief update visit or discussion with the Doctor, Specialist, or Nurse on the patient's present condition. With a proper explanation, this new approach worked well for both patients as well as the hospital financials and has now been in effect for many years. New initiatives such as "home delivery" of prescription refills by courier services was introduced and further improved on the process. This scheme proved particularly helpful to the elderly and those individuals with medical conditions requiring Caregiver support to move around. Further "home healthcare services" complement the process to distribute medications. Currently new software "applications" are under development to allow for ordering refills using a computer or mobile device to close the prescription refill process, yet keep costs affordable for all parties.

Additional initiatives to minimize "wastage" of drugs and medications that have been stored under controlled conditions, but when the "stock batch code" is nearing their designated expiry dates and the quantity on hand is too great, attempts to exchange the medication with another healthcare facility's Pharmacy where use of the drug is in greater demand, or failing which, the Chief Pharmacist may work with the Drug Distributor and request for testing of the medications stock batch and obtain a revised expiry date. Both those approaches allow for improved management of the medications as well as engaging Hospitals Pharmacy Departments and Healthcare facilities to work together and establishing an active "network" to be able to provide cross coverage support. This approach works very well, particularly on week-ends, holidays, and when there are periodic outbreaks of certain medical conditions, e.g. HFMD, SARS, various strains of bird flues, dengue, etc., creating spikes in usage, and an increased demand of certain drugs and medications. The important lesson learned is to be connected, by developing working relationships with Hospitals, and Healthcare facilities within your geographic area/ region. Remember, in times of emergency, coordinating services even with your "competitors" can become your best option as everyone is ultimately concerned with helping the patient. We must never forget that principle.

40 One must be able to understand and then explain the rationale **why Doctors/Specialists appointments may be delayed in their Scheduled Clinics,** despite their best intentions, as this question will be raised many times by individuals who believe Specialists are insensitive to their (patient's) time needs and write into the facility, local media, or other regulatory bodies to express their frustration, seeking relief.

It is both an accurate perception and fact that many Doctor and Specialist consultation appointments are delayed, some by a few minutes and in other instances as long as an hour, or more. Hospital and Healthcare Center Specialists have three distinct Service functions they perform – Conducting Ward Rounds, Performing Surgeries and/or Special Treatments, and providing access to medical attention via Specialist Outpatient Clinics (SOCs). Normally certain days and times are allocated to surgical and specialized treatment functions, and Scheduled Clinic Operations, while Ward Rounds will occur at least once, or more, every day.

40.1 Ward Rounds relates to the Specialist physically observing the patient, reviewing their overall medical condition by reading the documented "Progress Notes" from Nurses and other professionals (Pharmacists, Therapists, Radiologists, Pathologists, Lab Specialists, Dieticians, etc.) serving the patient. The Specialist's patient was admitted to hospital for a specific medical/surgical reason and they should be either recovering and improving as planned, or perhaps, incurring some planned or unplanned complication which needs immediate remedial attention that can be as simple as a minor change of medication, or treatment plan, to slightly more interventional actions, all the way to a radical change such as requiring immediate surgery or special treatment e.g. chemotherapy. If a serious enough complication occurs it may require even more time to organize the next course of action resulting in delay, affecting commencement of the scheduled Clinic time.

40.2 Surgeries and Special Treatment Sessions relates to the day(s) and time allocated to perform planned surgeries and treatments, but at times the schedule can be interrupted to perform emergency surgeries or treatments on patients who may be facing life-saving situations. This intervention, or a complication arising from a scheduled surgery, can either delay or postpone procedures. If a Clinic Session is scheduled AFTER the surgery or treatment time allocation, then there could be a delay.

40.3 Operating Clinics again are planned in advance on certain days; however. Clinic Sessions are the most flexible of the three key Service components provided by Doctors, i.e. managing Patients in hospitals, performing surgeries and/or active treatments. As patients are ambulatory and in most situations are not facing life threatening conditions, adjustments can be made. As a result, it is the Consultation Appointment Sessions that receive the bulk of complaints about delays. Interesting to note that in some instances a patient will experience a severe condition (collapse, AMI, respiratory conditions etc.), that can cause a delay for the remaining patients in the Clinic, to even the Clinic is not immune to delay once it is in session.

Besides Specialists being delayed due to evolving patient conditions in hospital, or while providing active services (surgeries, treatments), many patients also contribute to delays, such as,

40.3.1 Missing, or forgetting an appointment. This causes for alternative plans to be made. Over time, Clinic Staff gather enough information to determine an average length of an appointment, and then schedule appointments accordingly. At the same time, data is gathered on the number of "no-show" patients, and the number and amount of time is factored into the scheduling algorithm. However on certain days, ALL the patients will show up for their appointments on time, and this will cause a delay for the day, often at the expense of the Specialist and nurses sacrificing their lunch or break times to shorten the wait.

40.3.2 Arriving late for their appointment. When an appointment time is provided, the patient should arrive early enough to allow for a proper registration if it is for the first consult, or early enough for subsequent consults where any tests required can be completed in preparation for the Consult. Arriving at the exact appointment without making allowances for the preparation time required will cause a delay. In the meantime, other patient(s) will be managed, and you will wait.

40.3.3 Additional consult time. In many instances the patient will engage the Specialists with additional questions about their present condition, or even a new condition that may be identified by the Specialist requiring attention. The patient wants to ask additional questions of the Specialist while they have their attention. Another cause for an extended consultation time is when the patient or caregiver experiences difficulty in understanding the medical instructions being given by the Specialist, requiring more time of the doctor. However, in most cases the Nurses assist by continuing reinforcing the explanations outside of the Consultation Room to allow for another patient to be treated. Again, the additional time consumed can cause the consult time to be extended, and contributing to the backlog.

The Specialists are managing the needs, conditions, and expectation of all their patients who have been scheduled during the course of the day in one of their three Service areas, so the important "take away" of this long commentary is to ask the person raising the question if their perception would change "if it was them (or a member of their immediate family) who was in hospital, needing emergency surgery or special treatment, or experiencing a complication requiring the Specialist's attention, thereby causing other patients to wait while they are attending to you; or having the Specialist spend time explaining a certain medical condition you have while in the Clinic, taking longer than the allotted time; would they appreciate the time taken to treat them, or would they be satisfied with a strictly regimented Consultation that is concluded once the allotted time is up?"

Efforts have been made to minimize unnecessary waiting, and need ongoing attention. These efforts range from periodically updating the "average length" of an appointment consultation, and adjusting the appointment scheduling algorithm accordingly; building in one or two "empty" appointment times in the schedule to provide a "buffer" time to "catch up"; ensure a nurse is circulating and providing updates on any potential delays; and offer to reschedule or allow the patient "to be treated" by another doctor or Specialist with similar qualification who may be available. At many Hospital and Healthcare facilities, various instructional TV programs are aired to ease waiting time as well as having TV monitors dedicated to display your appointment number at various locations within the Facility, so patients can move around, or visit the garden, etc. Finally, many new computer and mobile Applications are being developed allowing for "on line" registration, and coordinated scheduling of required tests (Lab, Imaging, ECG, Stress, etc.) at a time before the initial, and subsequent appointments.

The same situation occurs in any Doctor or Specialist Clinic setting where an Appointment Model is used to facilitate scheduling Consultations for patients, whether in Private, or Government related Specialist Outpatient Clinics. Treatment in "first come-first served" or "triage" models follow different scheduling patterns.

The irony is, that patients are willing to wait, however long, to be seen by a Specialist who is considered to be "top" in the field, with no complaints (verbal or written) over either the wait or the fees.

41   One must **exercise caution and constraint** when criticizing One's predecessor(s) unless aware of **ALL the facts, details, and reasons surrounding previous actions and decisions taken (or not taken).** Conditions, such as internal management direction and/or Company political climate may have changed, so it is professionally prudent to project a positive and constructive attitude, following the principle of **continuous improvement** based on current management direction. Remember, one day, someone will succeed you.

As a newly appointed Member of Senior Management, or other managerial position (Heads of Departments/Services), effort should be taken to understand the current situation, and not immediately conclude or project the previous Team or any Individual Senior Manager(s) were wrong in their management. Typically, when new Individuals are appointed they serve a "honeymoon" period of 6-12 months in which Senior Management and/or the Board will indulge the new Individual(s) with financial, manpower, and operational support to implement change into the existing structure with a view for improvement. At the end of the "honeymoon" period the same Senior Management (Corporate HQ and/or the Board) will start to tighten the purse strings, and/or raise the "performance expectation bar" to cause the Management to become as efficient as possible. Initiatives for tightening of purse strings can come directly from the Board, various Ministries, or other key external sources providing funding, and key stakeholders in response to their objectives, as well as, responding to external economic conditions such as a downturn in the local, regional, or international economies which tend to run in cycles. Various practice and referral patterns due to technology, alliances, or Clustering can also change over time which will impact performance and workload statistics, thereby requiring management to review their priorities and realign them to the changing conditions.

Since this process occurs whenever there are changes to key Senior Management staff, one must understand the history of the activities that occurred and the actions taken. When there is a budget tightening, one of the first areas addressed is manpower, resulting in a reduction of staff; however, the work performed by the expanded staff acquired by the new management Team or Individuals will need to be reassigned to the remaining staff, downsized, or eliminated. The organization will go through many cycles over a period of years, while the internal tasks are continuously re-prioritized based on the latest Facility/Organization, or Corporate focus. Therefore what new Team Members or Individual will observe is only the "end result" of numerous adjustment cycles at a "point in time", which may give an incorrect perception. It is important to explore and understand both the clinical and financial contributions made by the organization, and what were the expectations of Corporate HQ or the Board at that time. One must know the history, so rash decisions or judgements should not be taken which could undermine the current status of clinical, operational, and financial performance to meet the key metrics.

So the best approach for the new Team or Individuals to take is review the current situation, look for areas where improvements, e.g. tighter compliance with established Policies and Procedures, and/or current Corporate or Board mandates, and make initial proposals on that basis. Ask the correct questions!

Remember at some point in time, your individual tenure and that of your Team will be over, and all will be replaced by another new Team, and the cycle will be repeated. Again, the new Team or Individuals will only "see" your performance at that "point in time", and you will be measured by the new Team's "perception yardstick", so how will you wish to be remembered? Therefore, be careful about assigning blame too quickly, and take a positive approach of "continued improvement".

42   Remember to **document discrepancies in key information and numbers submitted for budgets, reports or information,** as well as, any subsequent clarifications made, changes or corrections necessary based on reviewed information. Never consider the situation closed based on a telephone, or verbal discussion.

Failure to properly review any printed version of information submitted for consolidation while still in "draft" form to ensure it contains the same information as submitted, either by line item or in total, or failure to document in writing any approved subsequent changes or assumptions after a verbal discussion/ conversation over the phone or in person can have devastating implications when you may become the individual liable and responsible for the final outcome should there be a material difference, normally negative.

Therefore, **always request for and review information submitted** for inclusion in external reports after it is consolidated and attributed to you as the source to ensure accuracy of the information and that it is the same data and information submitted. There are times during the consolidation process, information is changed or modified, and if you do not seriously review the information, you will be accountable once the document is finalized, acted upon, and published or presented.

For example, you reviewed, approved, and submitted a budget for a particular program or project to individuals responsible for consolidating similar budgets from other Departments, or Facilities. Normally, you can ask for, or will receive a draft of the "work in process", and when received, take time to compare and validate the numbers or data to ensure they match what was submitted. If they agree, no further action may be required other than confirmation. However, if any figures, descriptions or key information has been changed or omitted, and you identify the difference(s), you should initiate verbal communication with individuals involved in the consolidation, and then ensure there is a documented "paper trail" in writing (letter, memo, email) reflecting your observations and potential implications/ concerns, or summarize key points of any verbal discussions or assumptions agreed upon. Without that paper trail, and depending on the materiality of the change in funding or content, should the changes not be made and there are negative consequences, you may be the individual held accountable, and the "penalty" will be proportionate. Regardless of how well you know the current individuals and can trust them, never presume they will be around in the future, and without the documentation, you have no evidence to protect yourself, and your career.

So, always take time to check any information submitted to other individuals responsible for consolidation, and document any discrepancies.

43   Whenever having documents translated, ensure the person performing the translation or reading the translated text is **knowledgeable in healthcare terminology**, and understands the nuances.

This observation may seem intuitive, and "common sense"; however, there are many instances where words and text are incorrectly translated, rendering the translation useless and potentially dangerous if followed. This principle is relevant in translations from your language to another, and vice versa. The individual who translates or reads the translated text must be familiar with medical terminology, and the context in which it is used. For example, in a Policy and Procedure for treatment of an adult patient with a particular medical condition, the term CRIB was used, which as a medical term means, "Complete Rest In Bed". When translated by an individual not familiar with medical terminology, the translation came out that the adult patient must be accommodated in a "crib", which is a baby bed! CRIB can have many meanings based on context it is being used, but only a few with medical interpretations; hence the importance of the nuances.

So, when having documents, instructions, books, P&Ps/SOPs, signage, media releases, Conference/Seminar promotional material translated make sure to have individuals versed in medical terms read all translations to ensure the interpretations are correct. It will save much in embarrassment.

44 It is an experience based observation - When transferring money to/from other countries, the **transaction's exchange rate received will usually be the most unfavorable** of the day.

How many times have you had to transfers funds for business (International Letters of Guarantee, International payments for supplies and equipment, sponsorship stipends, conference fees/applications for one or many attendees, etc.) as well as personal (mortgage payments, income tax payments, etc.) only to learn that the financial transaction occurred at the most unfavorable exchange rates of the day, thereby resulting in spending more than planned. While these are "costs of business" most financial professionals like to learn they have saved the organization money, regardless of the amount. Obviously, the greater the payment, the greater the impact of the unfavorable rates will be, but the feeling of the senior finance staff is that one has "lost" in the competitive battle of foreign exchange rates.

45 Developing a **credible Financial Model for a Feasibility Study** is a function of utilizing accurate

assumptions, facts, and statistics that can provide a defensible "anchor", and serve as reference points, able to be validated by both the Providers of the Financial Model as well as interested individuals and organizations reviewing the document as potential Investors, or Lenders.

Whenever a major project is under development, ranging from designing and development of a new hospital or healthcare facility, a major expansion of any existing facility, or introducing new programs, the key element is the provision and development of a credible Financial Model (Pro-Forma) and Feasibility Study, with sufficient insight, investigation, knowledge of economic, physical design, terrain and location, population demographics/profiles, existing competition, and legal /regulatory requirement to justify the assumptions which become critical considerations to the organization's bankers, shareholders, and stakeholders who will potentially be making an investment in the project.

A comprehensive Feasibility Study for a new hospital or facility is usually the most expensive pre-development component to complete, both from the actual Study up front, and could be the most expensive to all investors if the Project fails to achieve its objectives over time. Therefore, it must be done correctly with the most accurate information available, and built on defensible assumptions which make sense to the Owner, Developer, and Operator of the facility. Further, the Financial Model should be designed so it can be "flexed" in response to changes that may occur over the course of development planning. Assumptions made should serve as "proxies", and efforts should be made to "triangulate" and validate information used, both from "industry standards", and market research. The better the quality of information used and validated the more credible and defensible the numbers will be. Keep in mind potential Lenders and Investors will perform their own "due diligence" and will engage professionals to test the assumptions, looking for weaknesses in design and logic to challenge the basis. The better the information, the greater the likelihood the Pro-Forma will pass scrutiny, and give confidence to the potential Investors, and Lenders.

One common mistake often made is for an interested party (potential Owner or Developer) to decide they want to build, a hospital, medical center, clinics, etc. and decide they will spend "X" for the land, and "Y" dollars for building facility, equipment and operations without proper consideration on the scope of services and objectives. Once defined, the services to be provided, level of care to be given, and equipment required will define the quantum of resources to be sourced. Without the proper planning sequence, efforts are then taken to justify and make the hospital fit the expected investment size before ever doing the necessary Feasibility Study to learn whether it is justified. This results in a "cart before the horse" approach to develop the Project. However, it is important to note that in certain instances the idea of a hospital or healthcare facility may have merit, but the "timing" of the Project is too early, i.e. area will still need a certain number of years to reach the "tipping" point when the Project can be justified. In these instances, alternatives available are to defer the Project, scale back the concept and develop a service that can grow as the community grows, work with other existing facilities, or buy an existing facility. All are potential options!

While a Feasibility Study for a hospital (greenfield or brownfield) was used for discussion purposes, as it is the most comprehensive venture, the same principles and approach needs to be adopted for any major healthcare Project or Development. NOTE: Another important point to remember - when preparing the Financial Worksheet(s) Model (Pro-Forma) is to project "activity" over a ten to twelve year period of time forward to capture both the initial operational build-up costs, as well as time based facility renovations (7-10 years in the future), equipment replacement/upgrades, inflation, and projected "cost of capital" to allow for tracking, measuring, and analyzing EBITDA for the Project, which should be improving every year.

The Owner or Developer must perform their "Due Diligence" to determine the feasibility of undertaking the Project as there is substantial responsibility and financial exposure involved. It is more prudent to defer a decision to move ahead with the investment until after a properly prepared Feasibility Study is conducted, which addresses all the relevant questions, becoming the basis for a series of "workload drivers" and financial assumptions. Treat the cost of the Feasibility Study as an "insurance policy" to ensure decisions are taken with the best, most current information.

46   **When requesting a pricing related decision for approval**, ensure sufficient information is provided to take a decision, so include, incremental revenue, workload projections, costs (manpower, supplies/consumables, equipment (depreciation/amortization)), facility expenses, overheads, margins, and market assessment.

In a hospital or healthcare setting periodic pricing adjustments will need to be made to the published prices. If initially done correctly, performing a revision can be relatively easy. A general "rule of thumb" I always use is to perform a detailed costing every two years, with an interim inflation based adjustment (raise, retain, or reduce) in alternate years if economic and market conditions justify. When undertaking a pricing review, make sure all the key assumptions related to incremental revenue, workload, as well as operational and fixed cost expenses, and impact of changes in governmental policies and regulations are considered. Make sure basic assumptions are still valid, as workload (both increases and reduction) can change over time resulting in lower or higher cost per unit, as well as new products which can be either more, or less expensive. One other element to always consider is the gathering of current "market prices intelligence" for the same service from the competition or identification of general trends to ensure prices are reasonable. One must ensure you are comparing "apples with apples". Oftentimes, services in healthcare may have the same/similar names, but are "bundled" together (or unbundled), and the price captures the costing and pricing for the bundled services, so ensure the product/services are the same, lest your prices appear to be too low or too high. If necessary, change your description to reflect any uniqueness of the product/service to justify the specific pricing. A good example is the Daily Room Rate (DRR) which is normally a "published rate" and is used to make quick comparisons between hospital prices easier. Most DRRs are comprised of three basic components: cost of the bed (facility and equipment related); cost of basic nursing/medical services (depending on the intensity of care required, e.g., ICU, "stepdown/progressive" care, general medical and surgical wards "lying-in" wards inclusive of floor medications; and, cost of food. In some markets, Hospitals try to be creative in marketing and take advantage of potential patients/customers naiveté about the services included, and split the DRR into the three components with separate charges, i.e., Room, Nursing, and Food. Looking at only the "unbundled" Room Rate charge, it will create a market perception that the cost of services at the particular hospital with be more favorable than an alternative Hospital, when in fact, if the fees for the components are combined, the resultant DRR Fees would be comparable, or even more than the traditional method of representing the Daily Room Rates. So be mindful of this practice, and be sure to include a brief description of the components provided in the marketing material.

Another meaningful example is pricing of Imaging Department services, as they tend to be market driven, and may not be reflective of actual cost recovery for the service provided. While this is an established practice, ensure your pricing review takes this into consideration and adjust accordingly to be competitive. Certain imaging services can enjoy a higher mark-up over cost recovery for the services provided based on the latest technology, while more established procedures using lower end technology may be priced below actual costs due to the competitiveness. Also remember, cost recovery is a function of the direct cost of equipment, achieving near optimal utilization (volume and time), and related direct and indirect overheads.

The points to remember are: be knowledgeable on your costs; be flexible; be proactive; and KNOW your competition.

47   **Staff must understand the need to be productive**, methods to measure productivity, and the minimal individual performance levels required which will collectively improve the organization with sufficient workload to financially survive, at an affordable price structure, to the population being served, and result in a good "value for money" perspective.

Regardless of whether your facility is a government owned or a private healthcare organization, there is the need to encourage staff to be productive, from the lowest level to the most senior staff, as each person contributes according to their role and responsibilities. Each facility should develop and adopt measurable workload metrics and productivity standards, so proper staffing ratios can be determined for optimal productivity. As manpower is the largest component in the organization's operating budget, judicious utilization of staff can make a difference between a profit/loss situation of the healthcare facility.

If Management is unfamiliar with target productivity numbers, an option available for hospitals and healthcare facilities is to engage "Industrial Engineer" Consultants to perform productivity analysis, using manpower time study techniques, which take into account established general industry standards, and modify them according to the unique physical and operational conditions of the facility, e.g. layout of wards, and technology level, e.g. use of computers versus manual processing of data, capturing services, or performing treatments and determine the staffing required to monitor and manage patient needs. Further, if the Healthcare Group is sufficiently large, the

Headquarters Division may establish a Department/Services to perform similar reviews internally.

Staffing and individual staff workloads can then be adjusted to meet changes for key variables related to treatment of patients, such as nursing patient-staff ratios by medical acuity of the patient, e.g. ICU, stepdown, lying-in ward, or number of nurse to doctor ratio in the outpatient clinic, number of lab tests, pharmacy prescriptions, imaging procedures per staff, or the number of Operating Room/Theatre surgeries that can be performed within specified period of times. There are many variable affecting productivity numbers, so it is important to identify the proper numbers, so workload and staff requirements can be achieved to take care of the patients. This is also applicable to operational support services areas such as the Kitchen/Dietary services, Environmental/Housekeeping Services, Medical Records, etc.

Department Managers must understand the principles of productivity and matching of resources to workload, and they should be able to calculate their staffing requirements based on the workload numbers and plan accordingly. Following this concept, the Managers can meet and operate within their budget parameters. One important item, is that areas where there is variability of workload, e.g. wards, OR/OTs, Clinics, etc., staffing should be designed with a mix of full time, part-time, "floating" staff, as well as access to "contract/temp" staff who have been pre-cleared, and can be engaged on short notice to meet the vagaries of seasonal workload dynamics and thereby avoid excessive, sustained overtime (creating risk of errors due to being tired), or under-utilized staff (who do not have sufficient work to justify their position).

Productivity must be inculcated into all staff, so they both appreciate the work they perform, and be proud of their contributions in serving the patients.

48. When evaluating acquisition of expensive equipment there are two primary methods of financing the purchases, either by outright purchase, or term leasing. **Always perform a "life cycle" analysis** between the two options taking into considerations of all related costs.

A financial exercise that should be adopted and used more frequently is the concept of "life cycle" analysis. The objective is to evaluate financing alternatives to acquire access to key and expensive pieces of equipment used for patient diagnostics or therapeutic treatment in the best manner to optimize cash requirements. It is primarily used for purchasing Imaging Department items such as MRI, PET, CT (and various combinations), Cath Labs, Linear Accelerators (LINAC), Operating Room/Theatre equipment such as Robotic or interoperative MRI, or entire package of equipment for a new OR/OT, as well as, IT hardware, software, implementation, and peripherals if acquired as a "package" from a vendor. Only once all the specifications and requirements have been defined, should the acquisition process commence.

The first Option is for outright purchase of the above items, either for new facilities, new programs, or replacement/expansion of existing equipment. The organization should obtain multiple competitive quotations for outright purchase of the equipment, plus related annual maintenance and upgrade costs of the hardware and software, after expiration of warranty, as well as quotes for supplies and consumables to support and operate the equipment, normally for a minimum combined period of five years. Using a projected number of procedures/workload over the five years, then the Finance Team can calculate the cost per procedure, which is critical in the final comparison analysis, and price setting targets for the services.

The alternative option is to enter into a long term lease/lease purchase agreement (either based on "fee per procedure, or fixed sum tiers) for the same equipment, having the same features as for the purchased items. The finance/lease arrangement should be designed for a period of five years, similar to the outright purchase analysis. In most cases the lease is for the equipment only and the supplies and consumables are charged at a separate, agreed upon rate structure. Agreements can be a "flat fee" based on time billing, i.e. every 90-120 days, or by per procedure. Again, have the Finance Team calculate the cost per procedure so the figures can be compared with the outright purchase profile. The quotes can be obtained from the same vendors as the "outright purchase" vendors as well as other vendors who wish to participate.

Once the calculations are performed and expressed in a "per procedure" basis, all the quotes meeting the specification requirements can be displayed in a spread sheet, and then the organization can take an informed decision on which approach to take. At times the results can be quite interesting and worth the time and effort to perform the "life cycle analysis".

Regardless of whether the hospital is private or government owned, this analysis can be useful in the selection process from the financial perspective as it also allows for planning of cash requirements, and cash flow. Obviously, if payments were made based on a per procedure use, normally with a minimum number for a specific time period, the cash flow is in better alignment with the workload, while the outright purchase typically requires all or most of the cash up front or in "progress payments". Once the numbers are finalized, the depreciation can be calculated and allocated over the useful life of the equipment. It can then be further allocated amongst the number of projected procedures per year. The Finance Team can help to perform this calculation. Once this is done, there can be some negotiation and fine tuning of terms and pricing to best meet the needs of the organization. While there will be interest payments associated with any lease arrangements, the amount of interest incurred would be taken into consideration for the opportunity cost and funds available for additional equipment, rather than a complete payment. There is still a variant on the cash payment mode, and that is where a component of the cash is contributed from the hospitals accumulated reserves, and another portion may be borrowed from a bank.

Note: In some Government owned and operated situations, a decision may be taken for the outright purchase option, as the Capital requirement amount may only be available in the current fiscal year budget, so the facility may be unable to "guarantee" or commit sufficient operating budget expenses for subsequent years using the lease approach. Obviously, this would influence the decision process.

The important point is to understand the concept, and perform the calculations to determine the arrangement that best meets the financial and cash flow needs of the organization.

49   Whenever you make a presentation, or deliver a paper, at a Conference/Seminar, **you learn more in the process** than you can actually convey in your presentation.

When asked to make a presentation on a specific topic at a conference or seminar, or presenting a research paper, I am always intrigued by the amount of information reviewed to make the presentation. Normally we will search the internet, visit a library, discuss the topic with other individuals knowledgeable to both expand our knowledge and develop a sense of what key points we want to convey, and people want to hear. In that process of information gathering, we learn more about the details and intricacies of the topic than previously understood. It is truly a learning experience, and cannot be any less intensive than writing or preparing a paper for a class in university. Part of the learning process is that it raises questions and issues which cause one to further investigate the causes and implications so you can answer any questions that may arise from the presentation. One must always anticipate questions from the audience during the Q & A segment of the presentation making certain observations or offering different views or comments which will challenge you as the presenter. A well prepared presenter will have considered most points, particularly if they are subjective and should be able to develop a reasonable explanation or justification should any position be contrary to the audience's perspective. Even if there is nothing contentious in the presentation, and you are already recognized as being knowledgeable (an expert) on the subject matter, "doing one's homework" when preparing the presentation is a fulfilling activity. Depending on the frequency of presentations on a particular subject matter, the knowledge base of the individual will continue to grow over time and be refreshed as one becomes more comfortable with the material, and more "expert" on the topic.

So it is a great learning experience as you prepare for a presentation. Remember, at most conferences and seminars the attendees will have paid (either directly or through sponsorship) to hear you speak, so one has the obligation to take pride in the presentation, "know the material" being presented, and make it a pleasant learning opportunity for the audience.

50   In preparation of slides for presentation, a good "rule of thumb" is to **allow each content slide one, to one and a half minutes**, so plan accordingly.

Over the years, having both participated in making presentations as well as having the opportunity to attend many others, I often calculate the average time of the presentation, by watching the start and ending times, and dividing the calculated time by the number of content slides presented. (Content slides equal total slides, less the introduction, agenda related inserts as one moves through the presentation). This number tends to be within the range of one to one and a half minutes for each content slide. Depending on how much experience one has in making presentations, this bit of information is useful in planning your content. It also allows you a simple way to determine the range of slides required for the specified period of time allotted for your presentation. So, for every 15 minutes of presentation time, allow for 10-15 content slides depending on the complexity of material being presented, and potential questions to be asked. After preparing the slides, using a stop watch, practice your delivery at least three to five times to determine if your presentation falls with the allotted time, and modify accordingly. Each time you practice, the delivery will become smoother, and more professional.

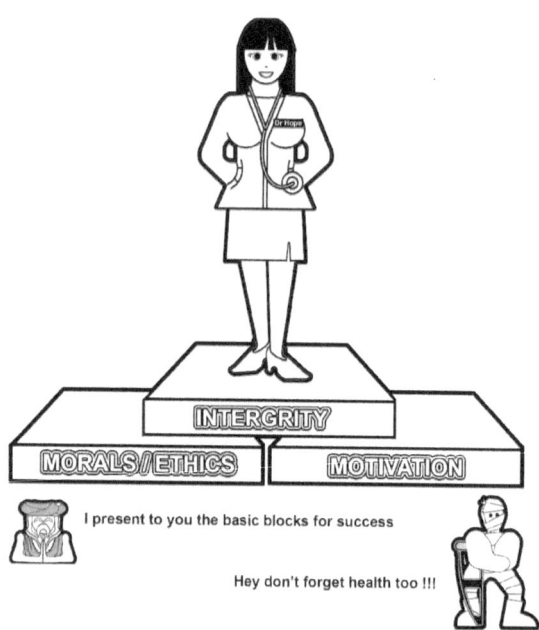

51 Remember, individual **integrity, motivation, and ethics/morals** are the building blocks of a successful professional, and cannot be taught. If staff demonstrate any lack or weakness of these characteristics during the probation period, then it is best for all to release the individual, as they could cause problems for you and the organization.

When hiring staff, regardless of level, one always tries to find the best "fit" for the position. At times there are instances when the ideal candidate cannot be found, so the next best option is to select the most promising candidate to be engaged, after a "due diligence" reference check is performed. Most organizational, operational, and educational shortcomings a potential staff may have, can normally be overcome with proper orientation, on-the-job training, and attendance at focused courses to mold the individual, develop their career path, and establish their worth. This is often the case when recruiting individuals fresh out of the education system, those "released" as a result of a downsizing exercise, coming from another industry, or military. Therefore, in the course of the resume reviews and face-to-face interviews with short listed candidates, one must look for any shortfall in integrity, motivation, or ethic/morals as individuals lacking these required personality attributes will be problematic. Normally they are difficult to impossible to change, so if any signs arise, it will be in both your, and the organization's best interest to "pass" on the individual, even if all the other attributes and skills are achieving a "green light".

Sooner or later, those personality flaws will emerge and create problems. The longer the individual(s) are with the organization, the more entrenched they become, the more difficult it will be to remove them. At first the shortcomings will be subtle, but over time more obvious. Regardless of the individuals position within the organization, evidence will need to be gathered and documented, counselling may be required to meet various workplace fair labor practice guidelines, requiring gathering of extensive documentation to build the case and protect the organization from any potential allegations of wrongful termination. If any of the attributes become apparent during the probationary period, do not confirm the individual, and in most cases, releasing them from the position should not be a problem. Obviously, if any of the attributes leads to fraud, theft or other serious organization defined breaches, then the individuals can and will need to be managed in the defined manner, as well as taking consideration if any legal or police action will be required.

The best approach is to be careful and ask good, probing questions to select the most promising candidates; however, if a problematic individual is hired, just be aware that it will take time to resolve the issue, and in the meantime, it may create morale, communication, and other supervisory issues with other staff. The higher the position the individual occupies, the greater the potential damage that can be inflicted and the greater amount of time required to rectify the situation.

52. For staff involved in "**sabotaging**" **one's peers or supervisors for the purpose of faster advancement, they will eventually be identified;** it is only a matter of time before corrective action(s) will be taken either directly or indirectly to remove them from the organization, as well as affecting their individual credibility, ethics, and integrity.

Unfortunately, there are instances when certain staff perceive themselves better than their peers, and plan to "move" up the career ladder faster than their peers with a view to even overtaking their immediate supervisor's position. Typically, they will collaborate with one or two other individuals (in the same or other departments) to create situations where "fake", or "taken out of context" information is presented as fact and used against their peers or immediate supervisor with the objective to discredit their work and have them removed from their positions, ultimately positioning themselves for an accelerated climb on the promotion ladder. The perpetrator and collaborator(s) will make a presentation to a more senior individual in the hierarchy who may not be aware of the details of certain operations, who then accepts the allegations as fact, and take decisions accordingly to the detriment of the staff and supervisor.

This approach may work for a period of time, but over time will cause the department or organization to develop internal problems that cannot be suitably resolved and kept "hidden". Oftentimes, the External/Internal Auditors are the individuals who serve as the catalyst to identify shortcomings and will raise concern with Senior Management about the quality of the financial accounts, or other observed operational shortcomings and highlight the need for rectification. If not already known, once the individual(s) involved are identified, Supervisors and Human Resource Managers will be tasked to take appropriate steps to release and replace the individual(s). Until such time that this occurs, the ongoing operations of the entity are at risk.

53 To be a good teacher (Supervisor, Manager, Mentor), **one must know what is right from wrong**, expected or unexpected outcome, principles and reasons for any action, procedures, surgery, or treatment and understand the process. This can only be learned over time through practice and performance.

More senior staff are often paired with new staff and tasked to be a "teacher/helper" to assist in daily operational development of staff; so, it is important that the teacher is familiar enough with the internal workings of the operations to orientate and educate. Most activities within the department or organization have a specific reason or purpose, so nothing should be done on "remote control" without understanding the purpose. A good teacher will understand the parameters or acceptable condition ranges, and can identify when certain results are "flagging" outside the normal range and requiring corrective action to be taken. An understanding of the underlying causes and ways to rectify the situation should be part of the training shared by the teacher while they activate the corrective plans and monitor the results. A good analogy would be a fuel/petrol gauge on a vehicle. It is always clearly marked when the tank is full or approaching empty, so the driver knows what actions need to be taken at either extremes. It is the same with financial, operational, and performance results. The experienced teacher can "read" the results (financial or operational metrics) and determine what is happening and if it is acceptable and inculcate these skills in their staff under training. If they cannot answer the cause of a situation, they must investigate and learn the reason, as a new concern or issue may be evolving which should be identified early. This practice will ensure the development of both the teacher as well as the individual being trained. A good, confident teacher will want to pass this type information along as they recognize they are not indispensable, and should something happen to the teacher, the teacher would feel comfortable and confident with their staff taking the necessary actions. Further, training subordinate or peer staff to learn the duties and how to manage different conditions and situations, places the teacher in a good position for promotion should an opportunity emerge, as well as the staff under guidance of the teacher in a position for serious consideration to fill the teacher's position.

54 **Climbing the career progress ladder too quickly**, particularly during good economic times, **fails to provide individuals with sufficient exposure, knowledge and experience** to manage difficult situations and/or required actions or different approaches to take during times of economic down turns.

There have been many staff who have worked for the organization for a short period of time, less than six months, who when offered a small incremental increase, or a fancier title will decide to resign from their current position. We may try to talk them out of the decision, but most time when the decision is taken, they have made their mind up to leave. It is important that whatever one's position in the organization may be, it is important to gain the necessary experience on how to manage the situation in both good and bad times, economic, or political times. Having a good teacher to work with, during both type cycles helps develop the individual's experience, character and understanding on what to do, and the potential outcomes to be achieved. It is much easier to survive in a growing, expanding market, where all the actions generate business, so hiring of staff, expanding programs are "happy events" from a management perspective. But what happens when there is an economic downturn? Every crisis or economic downturn will be different, so the actions taken in response may be developed based on previous experiences. The final solution to manage the emerging problem may be directly or indirectly based on prior experience. So, if a person has risen too quickly in the organization's hierarchy without gathering incremental experience and knowledge on how to manage in both good and bad situations, they will be at a disadvantage when a real crisis or severe downturn occurs.

My advice is to stay with an organization for a reasonable period of time (minimum six to twelve months, to learn about the different positions in the department or organization, their responsibilities, the roles they play, and the authority they have to influence change. Learn and work with your supervisor about how to manage a situation should one or more of the regular staff be off work for an extended period of time or the company has to "downsize" manpower because of a downturn in the economy, workload, or funding sources. Take time to discuss ideas about what might be the appropriate actions and options necessary to manage the situation, e.g. prioritizing tasks, distribution or reassignment of work/tasks, cross training staff, learn what operations can be streamlined, send staff for specialized training, consider short/long term outsourcing, engaging consultants, or other viable ideas. Learn to develop, grow and think (in or outside the box) ideas using experiences gained while under a proper supervisory structure.

The biggest concern for the individual should be their ability to manage operational situations in time of economic downturns resulting in downsizing of staff or operations. This type of situation will stress test the experience factor and performance ability of staff. Those with sufficient depth will succeed; those with insufficient exposure to operating under those conditions will either be demoted, resign or be terminated.

55 HR Departments should have a record of anyone who has ever been affiliated with the

Organization. Names of individuals provided by business partners, attachments, volunteers, students, etc. should be recorded for legal and insurance purposes, in the event a situation ever arises where there is a need to establish a relationship or connection. Outsourcing is a management tool/option, so organization's still have responsibility to keep a record as if staff were on payroll. Think, **Worker's Comp claim, theft (money, equipment, IP), fraud, recognition for an award, relationship with someone in the organization, etc.**

This concept of maintaining a record of all individuals who have ever worked for the organization, either on payroll, contract, volunteers, attachments, "partnership", or outsourced contractual "partnership" arrangement is difficult to be accepted by most Human Resource Departments (HRD). There is a perception that if any individuals are not on direct payroll (i.e., paid directly by the organization), the HRD is not required to maintain a record of their affiliation with the hospital, or healthcare facility. Often the rational given is that the sponsoring organization, "partners", contract staff employers, or any other source where the individuals came from, e.g. universities, trade/nursing/technical/specialty schools, would have a record of the individual(s) posted to the hospital or healthcare facility. However, that approach fails to capture the locations, dates, times and where the individuals were assigned, what duties given as this can affect potential work related injury claims which may not be lodged for an extended period of time, or for reference, referral purposes. The source providing the staff may only be able to acknowledge that the individuals were assigned to your organization, but as indicated, cannot attest where, what, and when they actually worked. Also, external organizations contracted to provide staff may not have their records, or even be in business when a need to verify someone's affiliation with the healthcare facility. Further, for security purposes, all authorized staff in the hospital or healthcare facility should be given proper identification badge, preferably with their picture, name, title, and a permanent or temporary ID Number. Staff should be encouraged to "challenge" anyone i.e. ask who they are, why they are in a specific location, etc. within a Department or "restricted area" especially if they are without proper identification or reason. If not satisfied with their explanation, a supervisor or security should be called immediately, and/or they should be escorted out of the immediate area.

56 **Never wait till appraisal time to counsel a staff for poor performance.** Do it as soon as a shortfall, or decline in performance is identified. Try to learn the cause, to both help staff, and try saving the work relationship, as well as your investment in developing the staff.

Whenever there is an obvious decline in a staff's performance, as a Manager, we should take the initiative to meet with the staff to learn what may be the cause, and look for ways to assist them, and salvage the individual's career. To allow the deterioration to continue is counterproductive to the organization as well as the staff concerned. NEVER wait until the annual appraisal time to raise any issues, as the staff will be surprised, and you will have contributed by allowing productivity and performance to decline which sends the wrong message to the staff. The best thing to do is meet with the staff involved, have a discussion and attempt to come up with a plan to continue being productive at work, and help the staff separate home related issues from work wherever possible. If not possible, then it is best to arrange for the staff to take time off to resolve their personal issues, or work with the Human Resource Department to assist in arranging professional Counselling. In most instances, you will have invested a substantial amount of time in training staff, a combination of both on-the-job and formal, structured training ranging from in-house or external training opportunities, so you want the staff to be productive and contribute in their roles.

So, be positive and take action when you either notice or are made aware of a staff with potential problems (either at work or home). Salvage the relationship, salvage the staff, and you will also be recognized as a helpful, caring Boss and Manager.

57   If and when managing a difficult employee, **prepare a detailed chronological record of actions**, conversations, observations, and feedback received to support any actions that may need to be taken.

Unfortunately there are instances where a member of senior management or manager level becomes problematic. This may be observed by lack of follow though in work commitments, lack of initiative, or alternatively taking more initiative than appropriate or authorized, failing to prepare and file mandatory reports, or other observed shortfalls in official protocol. Certain minor deviations in themselves may not warrant serious concern and could be innocent infractions; however, when a pattern emerges to a point where other staff have difficulty in working with the individual, or external parties pass comments back to management, something needs to be done. As a more/most senior individual, one must take steps to address the situation, lest other staff become frustrated, morale drops and they look to leave. This is not a healthy situation for either the Manager or Company. Normally as professionals, we should attempt to have a discussion with the individual involved, and bring the situation to their attention and the problems occurring. Should the situation persist, then it may be time to start documenting all dates and times of informal, then formal discussions, meetings/counseling, efforts, as well as topics discussed, guidelines provided, and establishment of a "work improvement" plan with a defined timetable, and measurable outcomes provided and agreed upon. It is now time to develop a chronology of events leading up to the point where a decision to terminate or part company with the individual is taken. The purpose is that as a professional, the individual may initiate certain actions after leaving the organization, or file appeals to more senior officials within the organization, all the way up to the Board Members, or even outside the organization, to Ministries/Departments to make a case for "wrongful termination". Without a clear documented chronology as the process unfolds, and without "evidence" with samples of shortfalls, and guidance provided to help the individual, the organization will be at a disadvantage in representing themselves. The documented chronology allows for sharing key information elements and establishing facts. While the argument could still be made that the employer is still biased, the documentation must show a pattern and actions taken. Further, when having to manage this type individual, it is also wise to periodically include representation from another senior individual aware of the situation or Human Resources

Department to participate, and listen to the situation, and offer an objective independent perspective and any idea(s) on how to salvage the situation. Unfortunately, if the situation has deteriorated to such a point, confidence, trust, and ability to work together will have been lost, so the best solution is normally a parting of ways, either by formal dismissal or allowing for an immediate resignation.

While an amicable agreement to part (usually voluntary submission of a resignation letter) may be a reasonable solution, it would be shortsighted to presume that will end the situation, as their failure to secure employment can result in individual blaming the previous employer, causing them to file a claim, or engage a lawyer to seek justice. Having the chronological record of action, feedback from other staff, documented examples, statements, complaints filed displaying the shortcoming provide a better basis for justification for the actions taken.

Therefore, it would behoove one to commence preparation of a record as soon as there are indications of non-compliance, and keep updating it until either the individual is able to resolve and comply, which is preferred, or other actions are taken. Sad to say, when this type situation starts to occur and not understood and rectified quickly, trust will be lost and the individual's promotional opportunities will rapidly decline, or generate a permanent record that will follow them throughout their professional career.

58   Effort should be made to **maintain contact with retired staff**, so that in times of emergency they may

be contacted, and can be reactivated to assist during times of emergencies.

In most instances when a staff retires from the organization, whether after many years of service and reaching mandatory "retirement age", or taking "long care leave" to look after a growing family, or serve as a caretaker of a disabled family member, or some other legitimate reason, the individual's personnel files and names are normally archived and dropped from the organization's records. On various occasions I have recommended that this "retired" group of staff be kept informed of activities via Newsletters given to active staff, and even invited to various hospital functions such as Family Day, Dinner-Dances, or other social events to maintain contact.

There are various reason this idea has been promoted which could benefit both parties. It –

58.1 Provides recognition to the individuals for their contributions over the years,

58.2 Offers the retirees an opportunity to network and keep in contact with friends and associates they developed over the years. The age related retirees can also feel lonely, isolated, and not a part of anything, and those who retired to take time to raise a family, or look after a disabled family member may appreciate maintaining contact as they may be available to work again in the future. If the hospital or facility needs such staff, re-engaging these staff could help to reduce recruitment costs and "fast track" training them again to become productive,

58.3 Provides access to a valuable manpower pool who could be contacted and mobilized during times of emergencies, or outbreaks. During the SARS epidemic, efforts were made to contact various doctors, and nurses to return to the hospital to help serve and assist in looking after patients, or other clinical administrative support duties to help the "front line staff" cope. They are already trained, and know the environment, so rather than trying to recruit staff to assist during this time which will be hard, the retirees can be engaged and mobilized, and appreciated.

So for the reasons cited, and there are probably more, serious consideration should be given to maintain contact with "retired" staff from your organization. In many instances the "retired staff" will not attend even if invited, but it would make them appreciative in the knowledge that they are or were valuable to the organization, and if a need ever arose, they would be more likely to be reactivated for a short period of time.

59 Promote **adoption of** and compliance with **professional Credentials, Operational Accreditations, Facility Design Standards,** and "best practices" which will raise the "real and perceived" quality of services provided by the hospital or healthcare facility; however they come at a cost, and the organization must be committed, to achieve the results.

As a current Senior Administrative decision maker (CEO, CMB, COO, CFO, CIO, CNO or equivalents) or a future one, at some point you will be approached, by developers, investors, owners to participate in strategies to either develop a new hospital(s)/healthcare facility, or as part of a "due diligence" Team appointed to evaluate an existing hospital(s) or healthcare facility for potential acquisition. Many decisions relating to adoption of and compliance with established professional Standards, and seeking Accreditation will need to be made. Each decision will have both an operational and cost ramifications to the organization, and ultimately will impact the efficiency, quality, outcomes, and perception of services rendered at the facility. The decisions to adopt organization wide Professional and Accreditation standards will impact on the potential outcomes, success, and legal issues (malpractice, and other failures) to be resolved. Success will be determined on which standards are adopted and implemented, as they will set the hospital or facilities apart from other hospitals in the area/region, make it attractive and a hospital of choice for Specialists, nurses, and other professional operational staff, and recognized by the community and potential patient/customers. Listed below are a selection of areas where decisions will need to be taken early in the design and planning stages for "greenfield" development, or review of features already in place, or not in place, for a "brownfield" acquisition.

- 59.1 Medical Staff (Specialists) – Decision on professional Standards and Credentials of Specialists to be granted admitting privileges. This could be limited to those with Royal College, or Board Certification affiliations; or graduation from certain recognized local, regional or International Medical University Degrees; or perhaps no formal credentials, but certain experience qualifications. Besides the Specialists, this will influence decisions on their equipment and staffing requirements in their respective specialties. Medical By-Law Standards will also need to be finalized

59.2 Nursing Staff – Decision on the mix of Graduate Nurses to be engaged, international staffing standards to be adopted for all the different wards and treatment areas based on acuity, as well as ongoing Nursing Education, and training requirements.

59.3 Medical Management – Decisions regarding the adoption of Joint Commission International (JCI), and/or other country specific developed standards for medical management; how many years to implement; clinician design; and documentation requirements.

59.4 Clinical Support – Adopting Accreditation standards for each of the clinical support services, specifically, Laboratory, Imaging, Pharmacy, Dietary, all of which have recommended staffing, quality, workload metrics, staffing ratios, and educational standards.

59.5 Support Services – Medical Record (Document Management) Clinical Coding and storage Standards, Food Services, Internal and External Transportation Service, Communications, Media, etc.

59.6 Facility Design and Layout - Design, layout workflow, floor loading, zoning, vertical and horizontal patient/staff/public/operational (AGV, supply and food carts) movement, lighting standards, external traffic routing (zoning), incineration/waste disposal movement within the facility, energy efficiency and consumption management, e.g. building orientation, natural light, double/triple glazed windows, double wall construction, etc.

59.7 Power/Energy Standards – Redundancy of power sources, generators, electrical system design standards,

59.8 Security – Design of security features to adopt standards to manage lockdown, people flow, access, parking, AV/CCTV and other systems

59.9 Environmental – Design and accreditation of building for environmental issues, e.g., rainwater harvesting, roof-top greening, lighting, collection of general, sewage treatment, biological, and nuclear/toxic waste management standards,

59.10 IT and Computer – Standards relating to design, location of primary and alternate server farms, different computer software systems and implementation, hardware system configurations meeting international standards, data collection (PDPA) compliance, billing and other clinical reporting requirements, etc.

59.11 Business Continuity and ERM standards – Adoption of established Principles and Guidelines for all components,

59.12 Human Resources – Engaging professional compensation organizations to develop competitive salary scales to be used in the healthcare industry standards and establish baselines and other salary requirement or packages.

59.13 Accounting and Finance – Adoption of a standard setting body, e.g., Financial Accounting Standards Board (FASB) or equivalent, following Generally Accepted Accounting Practices (GAAP) for recording and reporting, as well as, setting requirement of individuals with necessary Accounting or Financial qualifications. Further, audited historical performance and validated projected future performance (Proforma) must be validated against industry performance, metrics to establish credibility and determine validity of the information be evaluated.

Failure to identify the expectations early before construction or omitting requirements for acquisitions will eventually become a burden and cause operational and financial issues over the entire life of the business. Therefore as Administrators being engaged in building or buying over an existing facility, care must be taken. Patient lives are "at stake", and depending on the standards adopted, and followed, will determine the Board's, and Company's exposure (clinical, financial, reputational) if anything goes awry.

Adoption of Standards and Accreditations will cost money and require an investment, but it will make a difference in the success of the Project. Finally, if building a new facility, many items can be incorporated in the design with minimal incremental investment, for others they will require an investment (e.g. double glazing windows, certain "double" walls, roofs). For a hospital or healthcare facility acquisition, the list and cost of making improvements and rectification of "non-compliance" items to meet your defined standards, and accreditations can be a negotiating point in determining valuation and price.

Remember, be the leader who make wise choices, and decisions as you may only have one opportunity for a very long time.

60. Hospital or Healthcare Administrative staff should never lose their perspective, **they are in the organization to support the Doctors/Specialists,** Nurses, and patient facing staff. If ever there is a decision on time for meetings, or administrative work to be performed, if it can be done by the Administrative staff that should be the default position, and preserve the Doctor's/Specialist's time for patient treatment, and patient facing support staff for clinical work.

Whenever there is a "conflict" with a difference in perception on who should take on responsibility of certain tasks, I always have the Administrative staff ask the simple question "is this something we can manage"? If the answer is "yes", then by default the Administrative or Support Staff are to assume the task(s), without involving patient facing Clinicians or Nurses. Only in situations where clinical input and participation is required, such as documenting clinical/services treatments or required conformance with performance standards, should we engage the Doctors, Nurses, or other patient facing staff. NOTE: There are certain administrative and support duties that can be performed by the various medical department staff who are not 100% directly involved in patient facing duties who are classified as administrative staff e.g. Secretaries, Personal Assistants, Clerks, Administrative Assistants but who can be engaged to gather information, prepare reports, reconcile data, and analyze information on behalf of the Specialists.

Administrative and Support staff must remember their roles are to support the Doctors, Nurses, and other patient facing individuals who are consulting and treating patients. While administrative and support staff roles are to complement the clinical services, we must keep the roles in perspective. Without patient-facing clinical staff consulting, treating, or performing operations on patients, there would be no administrative roles to perform. Their time is valuable, and critical in performing their roles, so whenever new operational or administrative related functions or tasks emerge for implementation or resolution, Administrative and Support staff must take responsibility to access the situation, and determine which individuals or department are to be involved in satisfying the new requirements. In that process, efforts should be made to determine if there is any overlap with existing requirements and eliminate duplicate work.

Do not complicate the front line, patient-facing staff with duties that can be performed by staff with administrative or support role duties. Preserve and allow them to focus on patient care. Consider this simple analogy: Doctors (providing the "horse power"), pulling the Cart (full of Nurses and Clinical Support staff) who are supported by the Wheels (Administrative and other staff) to make the Team move together in the same direction.

COMMON SENSE RELATED OBSERVATIONS

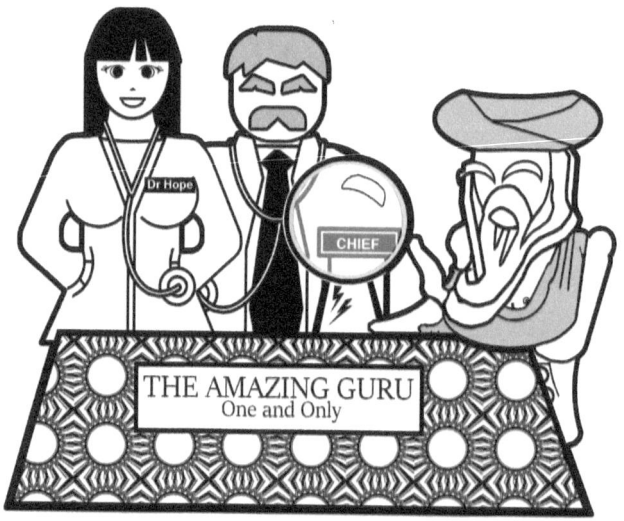

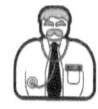 Why are we at the foretuneteller?
I asked for "common sense" not sixth sense !

1. Choose your friends carefully; otherwise there will be instances when you can say **"With friends like you, I need no enemies."**

When tasks need to be performed or responsibility given to achieve certain results, it normally requires cooperation, input and participation of many individuals working together, sharing of ideas, observations, and sharing suggestions to achieve the objectives. In most instances, key staff involved in the Project are required to make periodic presentations on Project progress to Senior levels of the Healthcare Management Team or Board Members. Should questions be raised during the presentation, all staff involved in the Project or assignment should be knowledgeable in the reasoning and actions taken, so they are consistent in their responses. However, there are instances when a Member(s) involved in Project/Assignment raise questions on actions or decisions taken (which should have been addressed in an internal discussion before the presentation) in front of Senior Management or the Board creating confusion and potential loss of confidence in the information presented. Normally the Project Leader or Members of the Team will respond and address any issue raised to maintain credibility and move ahead; however, subsequent feedback must be given to the staff who raised the question(s) that they created a "adversarial" position to what was being presented and discussed, which reflects poorly on the entire Team.

Any concerns a Team Member/Contributor may have regarding the Project or Assignment should be raised and resolved during the planning and implementation phase and not raised during any formal presentation. Hence, the feeling and basis of the statement "With friends like you, I need no enemies"!

The correct approach to be taken if an overlooked flaw or assumption does appear during the presentation is to pass a message to the Presenter, so they may clarify the results, or address the apparent shortcoming after validating the point subsequent to the presentation.

2   My grandfather used to say, "Sometimes, **other people are not as dumb as we are smart.**"

I initially learned this statement from my uneducated grandfather many years ago who dutifully took care of his family by working long hours in a factory. Over the years I have heard similar statements, but it took many more years to actually appreciate the significance of the observation. Often time we develop a perception that we are "so clever" having developed an idea that appears new and unique, and become a bit boastful, claiming ownership over being so inspired. However, when one looks at various practices in healthcare, in different locations and countries you will often find people doing similar things, perhaps with minor modifications and for a much longer time, that you believed you "discovered". This discovery then tends to bring reality to the individual, and puts their initial observation in perspective. Many times situations arise when substantial effort is made to close gaps and/or loopholes, applying different ingenious security and operational measures that are put in place only to learn they have been circumvented and neutralized by other individuals who developed the same observations of gaps and generated their own "solutions". So it is important never to become too over confident in what you do, but be humble and professional, and never underestimate creativity of others.

3   Always **keep your CV and Profile updated** and ready to use for professional reviews, Projects, reference, and career advancement opportunities.

Having a Curriculum Vitae (CV), or Resume, prepared and ready at all time is good personal internal planning. A properly prepared document should capture the essence of what transpired in various appointments throughout one's career, and should be reviewed and updated (rewritten, reformatted, lengthened, or shortened) at least once a year or whenever there is a change of employment. The purpose of keeping the CV/Resume current is not only to be able to produce it on short notice when required for a potential job opportunity for yourself, but also available to present "one's credentials and qualifications" when promoting or representing yourself for special projects being sought by your employer. For important Projects, financial and other key supporters being approached to make investments want to know, who and the "history" of the key individuals involved in the project, hence the CV is very important to provide the confidence and develop name recognition. With proper presentation, the probability of the company being "shortlisted" and potentially selected is greatly improved.

The Profile is a condensed version of the CV/Resume, with specific information extracted and designed to highlight relevant work experiences and skills for a particular project. This "snapshot" of your key qualifications is useful for presentations, introductions, and preparing submission documents such as Tenders, Feasibility Studies, Audits, Operational, and Financial Reviews. Therefore, it is beneficial to have multiple Profiles available to be used in the correct situation.

If managed properly, maintaining a CV/Resume and Profile will involve time with many reiterations, so it best reflects your professional career.

4   **Books you purchase** will more likely be read than those given for free.

Have you ever noticed how many books you have received and collected over the years as gift, or for attending a Seminar or Conference? They may have been included in the price of the ticket for the event, or given as "autographed" copies at the event, but they are a take-away from the event. Have you ever "taken stock" on how many you have actually read over the subsequent days or months? Most likely they nicely line your bookshelves and look impressive, but much of the information remains within the book covers, never explored or read.

On the other hand whenever you scour the bookstores for material, for either clinical, business, or professional related topics (accounting, customer, finance investment, management, marketing, medical, nursing, public relations, etc.) where you have a real professional need, or just for a "good entertainment read" by your favorite author(s), and you buy the book, there is a very high probability that you will read the book in part or total, maybe even more than once!. Sometimes, you may only read part of a business or technical book (a good example is "Idiot's Guide to/for something" series), it is probably due to the fact the book has many chapters or sections, And you may only need information about a specific topic at that time. This is fine as the book actually resolved your issues, and subsequently becomes a good investment and reference source.

Therefore, back to the opening statement, most instances book(s) purchased are read versus those received for free.

5   The grass is not always greener on the other side, **sometimes it's burnt**!

This simple alternative perspective to the statement of the "the grass always greener on the other side" suggests that all is not what it may appear to be and may only be a limited view of what a new situation or opportunity has to offer. There are situations where due to timing, opportunities will emerge that one could benefit both from a financial and experience perspective. In many instances, individuals only "see" the positive outcomes, without relating to the large amount of investment to be made in terms of time, effort, responsibilities, and other personal sacrifices required achieving the perceived rewards and experience. To reap benefits, one must also understand the correct mix of attitude, education, experience, commitment and teamwork plays.

At times the "grass is burnt" when after one makes a career/position change only to learn that the new position requires substantially longer hours to achieve "difficult, and sometimes seemingly impossible stretch targets", with all the stress and potential burnout associated. The levels of stress and challenge can be managed for a period of time; however, those who fail to have the commitment, physical, psychological, or emotional stamina will eventually give up. So, one trades off a currently good and known situation, for a potentially more rewarding opportunity by only looking at the "advertised outcome" possibilities and failing to appreciate all the efforts and demands required. Therefore, before making any serious career move, make sure the opportunity is aligned with your personal goal(s) and you have the necessary inventory of education, experience, to "value add" to the new position.

6   **A neat and tidy work area that is clear and clean projects efficiency**; whereas, a work area that is cluttered gives the impression of lack of organization and being behind schedule.

At various times we have a perception that all the piles of documents we may have on our desks and trays portray the level of activity we are involved and the amount of work we perform. However, I find that a long term buildup of documents, reports, etc. residing on the desktop actually reflects a potential backlog of work, which could cause delays and disruptions within the organization. Further, at times documents manage to "get lost" in the stacks and "no value work effort" is required by you or others to search for or reproduce the missing document, (I KNOW it's here, somewhere!) when it comes time to address the actual work. Therefore, a less cluttered or clear desk connotes an organized individual who manages workflow, and delegates in a more efficient manner. A good practice to adopt is every week or two to dedicate time and examine all the documents that have managed to accumulate, act on them or throw them away as the urgency or issue may already have been resolved pending your reading and taking action. This practice reduces documents as well as facilitates finding those that really need attention. At times, a delay in acting on an issue allows time for additional information relating to the issue to be collected which helps resolve the situation. Once the documentation is no longer required, file if important, or purge them in favor of clearing up the desktop. Being neat and tidy does not always infer a completely empty desk top, but rather one that is organized, so one can efficiently find the required documents.

7   Always be wary when things (benefits, opportunities, results being promoted) appear too good to be true.... **THEY USUALLY ARE!!!**

This caveat has been around for a long time, but is especially relevant to the healthcare industry. There are individuals, companies, organizations who promote use of their products to achieve "miracle" recoveries and substantially improve the "quality of life" for patients under treatment as either inpatients or outpatients. Patients are vulnerable, as they want to believe there may be cures or treatments that will shorten a treatment time/cycle, speed recovery and permanently improve their condition. However, one must be careful in management of patient expectations, and direct them to qualified clinical practitioners who are knowledgeable in a particular medical specialty. With the internet, people are able to research their conditions, and look for any promising treatments, but before general adoption, the treatments, products, supplements must be validated (clinical trials, studies, tests, and FDA or other government approvals) with regards to their efficacy before use.

Often patients and families will pose these type questions to the Clinical and Nursing staff attending to them, or even staff from the Quality Service Manager Section. So it is important to LISTEN but not unreservedly agree with their conclusions, as this can cause the individuals to interpret your actions as support to justify an incorrect perception of potential outcome. Again, direct their attention or facilitate engagement of qualified medical staff to address the patient's concerns. We need to adopt, and encourage others to practice healthy skepticism, being practical, and objective in considering situations where promoted results appear to be too good. This same level of healthy skepticism of potentially "unbelievable" positive outcomes in other areas is also recommended. This may occur for business proposals, business opportunities, financial performance, investments, research outcomes etc. It is important to perform "due diligence" for all proposals, calibrate and triangulate results from different perspectives, to ensure outcomes are realistic. Contact individuals who have experience in the respective fields. If all the lights are "green", then it is best to approach with caution, and "invest" in a small position to validate performance and claims. If realistic, one can always increase their position. Be cautious!

8. If you always try to save the **BEST FOR LAST**, you may find that you may not **LAST** to enjoy the **BEST**.

A common phrase and practice used both at work and in a personal context where you "save" the best ideas, concepts, materials, food, or plans with the intention to implement or take advantage of them in the future. This is often done at a personal level when a gift has been given but stored away with the objective to take it out at some future date or event. We are all mortal and changes outside our control often happen both at work and in our personal lives, which will preclude your best intentions to implement new concepts or ideas, or use new technology, gifts, or travel. At work a change in leadership could prevent you from introducing your ideas, or at a personal level, illness in the family or death may prevent one taking advantage of best ideas and plans for the future. So the moral of this observation is to be proactive and implement good or great ideas before it is too late, and take time off for those needed vacations you have always wanted before your health or other life or business events interrupt your plans.

9 The likelihood of receiving an important **telephone call increases dramatically whenever you go to take a shower, go to the toilet**, or are otherwise indisposed, so plan accordingly.

Another one of the Murphy's Law Category observations is with regards to telephone calls. How many times have you waited for a call, or not waited and the moment you go to take a "biological/toilet break", whether at the office or home, the telephone rings, same with taking a shower/bath, or taking a quick lunch or snack. You manage to settle in comfortably and then the telephone rings. If serious, it is unavoidable, but in some instances the calls are "wrong", "sales calls", hang ups, or someone has certain problems and want a "lending ear" to listen to their woes. During this time you are uncomfortably standing around. The real calls may need to be addressed; however, it does not make the experience less troublesome.

So, if your position requires you to be contactable, to manage any situation in a timely, professional manner you need to have a mobile or wireless phone or device, which can accompany you to all your various locations. Alternatively you could "call forward" your calls, or activate the voice message feature, and indicated you will call back within a specific period of time.

    10   The **battery on your mobile phone always goes flat** when you are expecting or making an important call.

This Murphy's Law candidate relates to your mobile phone failing when it is needed. Often time we use our mobile throughout the day for short conversations; however, often it will be late afternoon or early evening when we receive a really important, but lengthy call. If we are near the office or home we may have access to a recharging point, but I find that in most instances we may be away from a recharging point such as in a meeting, traveling in a taxi or other vehicle, waiting in a queue without access to the battery pack to allow for the continued conversation after your phone gives a "low battery" warning and less than five minutes before going completely flat and disconnecting the call. (NOTE: Check this out in your area. Most new mobile phones now have a low battery feature. Enter a certain number to extend the battery power. Obtain the number from a relevant App based on the specific mobile phone brand).

When this occurs, it is frustrating, and the only real solution to address the situation is to carry an emergency "battery pack" (with related connection cable). They can be added to the briefcase or purse. For safety purposes, the Telco industry's recommendation is to avoid carrying any battery next to your body.

    11   **One should never complain about being given too much work....** or having a high workload, be

thankful. Start to worry, when you are not given any work, or the workload goes away!

There are times when we can be in a situation where we perceive ourselves being overwhelmed, many targets, and deadlines to satisfy, and having a sense there is too much work to do, "cannot see the light at the end of the tunnel" situation. Occasionally this situation becomes a reality when one or two staff (sub-ordinates, peers, or supervisor) become sick, go on leave, or resign and you must assume certain key duties, to ensure meeting company, corporate, legal, regulatory, or Board requirements.

While in the short term it may be frustrating, it is also recognition of your skills and commitment that you are entrusted to ensure work is being completed. When the situation requires taking on additional duties, the first action to take is to prioritize commitments, and develop a workable timetable to spend the necessary time to complete the requisite tasks. Even when several commitment or deadline clash, still review which will have the greatest impact or the highest level of reporting responsibility to establish the priority sequence. In the worst case, be proactive and contact specific recipient parties to explain the situation and seek an extension, or co-opt other staff to assist in providing the work, and most will be helpful. So the key is to "take charge" and manage the situation. You may even engage staff to assist in managing the workload.

What is more frustrating and serious is when you are familiar with the work, available to assist in taking on additional responsibilities, but are "overlooked" as a potential provider. If this occurs, it is usually a result of previous experience(s) where you may have failed to deliver results in a timely, accurately manner, or have displayed an unacceptable attitude to your superior or others who needed your support, thereby resulting in a situation where one is isolated. This is the worrying condition as it will affect your appraisal and long term employment opportunities. If you note this pattern, then it is incumbent you take the necessary initiative to discuss the situation with your supervisor, identify and resolve any concerns, and become "part of the team" again, or you may need to seriously start planning an exit strategy from the company.

12   The need to retire from work should not be dictated solely by the function of age, but rather **be a function of how both the mind and body/age can perform** the tasks required.

This is certainly an interesting situation. Much has been written about this topic, so this is more a reinforcement of an understanding and how can it be managed. It is becoming more accepted that the worth and contribution of an individual is not exclusively a function of age, so there needs to be flexibility in interpretation and administration of the legal guidelines. While government normally passes legislation that sets official "retirement" ages to manage the demographic profiles of the general population, and used for insurance and other benefits, we all know that everyone is different. There is nothing magical that you will perform any differently the moment to achieve the mandatory retirement age, versus the days or years leading up the retirement age. Further as long as the individual's mental faculties are functioning properly, they have a tremendous amount of organizational, technical and industry memory stored away in their head, which should be "tapped" to help the younger generations. Unfortunately, many new generation individuals believe they know better, and end up repeating the same mistakes from earlier generations or turn around and implement changes that were in effect 15-25-30 years ago. In our younger years, we learned much from the senior staff, who passed along experience and guidance, which we merged with our "fresh ideas and approaches", which shortened our learning curves, and we become a more proficient individual, faster.

In some countries, the mandatory retirement age can be extended from three to five years as long as the individuals can pass the necessary physical examination and are functioning well. This is a great first step, and more countries should adopt this practice. As long as the average lifespan of the population continues to increase, the mandatory retirement guidelines need to be challenged, reviewed and revised periodically, as well as the duration of post retirement employment contracts. We can look around in both the private and public sectors and find many great senior statesmen and business individuals who far exceed the official retirement ages while still being productive and contributing in their respective professional areas.

13   As one gets older, **when you wake up in the morning**, it is no longer considered just a "Good Day", but rather **a "Great Day"**!

If one enjoys their profession and work in healthcare or any other industry, their work provides satisfaction with a sense of accomplishment and contribution, so every day we wake-up in good health and able to go to work is the beginning of another "good day".

As we age, and we still have that same passion and commitment for what we have done for many years, then each day we wake up, still in good health, and able to contribute, upgrade having a "good day", to become a "Great Day", thankful to the Good Lord for the continued opportunity to contribute both at work and spend time with our families. So when someone asks about your day, say "I'm having a GREAT Day"!

Having the additional time is a precious gift, and allows us as we become the "older generation", to share and pass along as much of our experience as possible to the "next generation", such as information shared in this book!

Have a GREAT DAY! Have a GREATLIFE!

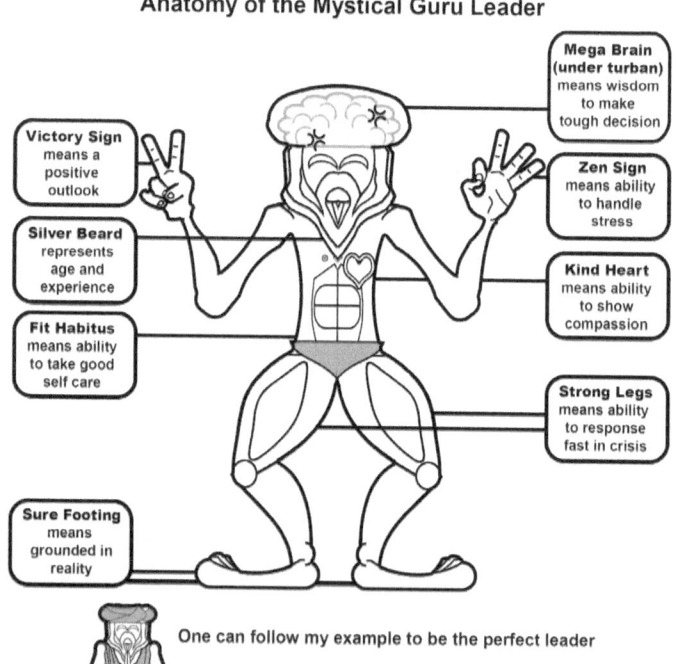

CLOSING

I hope you enjoyed the various Reflections and Lessons shared in this book. These are meant to enlighten and prepare you for many situations you may have to manage once you become a Manager or Administrator in a healthcare facility when interacting with patients and/or their families, or responding to internal staff, public, media, and legal queries. It is better to have thought about and understand some of the dynamics and background of situations that will occur and be prepared with rationale replies. In many instances, there are no "right or wrong" answers only approaches, and where there are no historical references, always look to your Guiding "First Principles" of doing "what is correct" to protect the lives and safety of your patients, your staff, you, and your organization. In many instances the examples and approach offered may only the "tip of the iceberg" and many other solutions are available.

Further, in complex situations, be professional and communicate with other knowledgeable staff within the organization, or if necessary, contact other professionals such as a Legal Panel (for legal related issues), Medical Associations and Ethic Committees (for Medical Issues), peers and other professionals at Department related Networks (Imaging, Pharmacy, Facilities, Security, Document Management, COO, CMBs, CNOs, CIOs, etc.) to discuss specific situations and solutions that can be considered. You are not alone! There is a wealth of experience "out there". This book tries to highlight many scenarios, and offer ideas that have been implemented, worked out, and considered as an access point to the creative thinking process. NOTE: Of course there will be the "nay-sayers", critics, and those who will not accept any explanation; as well as, those individuals who take advantage of the principles and systems and create embarrassing situations. Just do the correct thing!

As shared in the Preface, certain Reflections and Lessons appear obvious, and depending on both your maturity and experience within the Industry, as well as your facility, you may recognize some of situations being shared. You may want to use the book as a basis for discussion (with your Mentor or others) and sharing of ideas and approaches, and if the book helps to resolve an issue, or offer useful information to resolve even one situation, it will be worth the investment, and achieve the Author's objective, and being a Mentor.

SELECTED TERMS AND DEFINITIONS USED IN THE BOOK

Guru's Glossary of Selected Terms

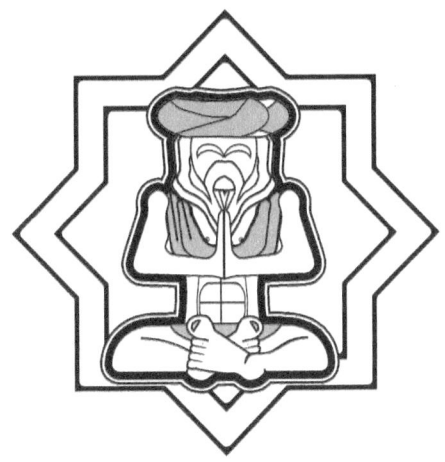

For those who desire more, I leave you with a glossary

Glossary: An alphabetical list of words and definitions relating to a specific subject with explanations

Acute Care

Care for conditions that have occurred due to a sudden event and are severe (potentially "life threatening") in nature. Services and treatments provided are intense and meant to stabilize patient's conditions and allow recovery.

Accident and Emergency (A&E)/Emergency Room (ER)

A 24 Hour Service available to manage real or perceived life threatening conditions by the patient, family, or caregiver. Normally having a separate entrance at a hospital, all patients will be "triaged" to establish their condition (requiring isolation) and severity to establish priority of treatment. A&E/ER Services (licensed by the Ministry/Department of Health) are one of the Medical Specialty Services provided by the hospital so if the patient's condition justifies admission, it can be arranged. If a patient's condition is more serious than the particular hospital can manage, the patient is given emergency care, stabilized, and transferred to another hospital able to treat the condition. Key features of an A&E/ER are:

1. Operational 24x7,
2. One or more Consultant Level Specialist's (normally Orthopedic or A&E/ER Trained) physically present to be able to immediately triage and manage trauma case (e.g. operate) and complex medical cases.
3. Supported with a Team of General Practitioner doctors, A&E/ER trained Nurses, and with,
4. Access to Lab(s), Imaging, and Pharmacy services,
5. Most A&E/ERs will also have a "medical observation/holding bay" with limited beds for doctors and nurses to observe certain patients, for up to eight hours should their conditions require,

6. Officially recognized A&E/ERs will also be part of any Emergency Ambulance Services network operating in the area,
7. Special License from Ministry/Department of Health

Ambulatory Care

Health related services rendered to persons who do not require admission and remain in a health care organization for less than 24 hours. Ambulatory Care individuals are often managed in "outpatient", "day surgery, ambulatory care centers" and Emergency Departments/Clinic service areas.

Ambulatory Services

The essential characteristic of "Ambulatory Services" is that the patient presents themselves, or is brought to the hospital or clinic for a purpose other than planned admission as an inpatient. Ambulatory services include Outpatient Services e.g., hospital based and/or free standing General Practitioner (GP) and Specialist Outpatient Clinics, Health Maintenance Organizations (HMOs), Poly-Clinics, 24 Outpatient Emergency Services, clinical support services, ambulance services, day surgery/treatment, and in-home health care services, etc.

Allied Health Services (AHS)

A cumulative group name of professional services available to assist the doctor in both their diagnostic assessment process and therapeutic treatments as part of the patient's on-going recovery. Examples of key Allied Health Services Departments are: Imaging, Laboratory, Pharmacy, Rehabilitation Therapies (Physical, Occupational, Speech, and Respiratory), Medical Social Work, and Dietary Counselling including all their detailed Department specific services/tests/procedures they perform.

Ancillary Services

Cumulative group name of services that support front line service providers, e.g. doctors, specialists, nurses, etc. by providing the necessary infrastructure to facilitate management of patients. Examples of key Ancillary Services are: Outpatient Clinics (Outpatient, Endoscopy, Ambulatory Care, etc.), Medical Records (Document Management), Patient Transport Services (Internal and External), Appointment/Call Centers, etc.

Automated Guided Vehicles (AGVs)

Vehicles, flat and heavy in design, battery powered, automatic, and responsive to electronic instructions to transport carts of items (patient food trays, medical records, fresh laundry/linen, prescriptions, etc.) from a particular department to another without manual intervention. They are programmed to "call" for a dedicated AGV lift, which provides vertical movement for them. Their route follows imbedded metal strips located under floor covering to arrive at their designated destination where they wait until released to return to their primary location.

Average Length of Stay (ALOS)

Average length of stay is the average number of patient days of service rendered to inpatients during a given time period. It can be calculated by either using Total Discharge Patient Days/ Discharges; or, Total Patient Days/Admissions for a specific period of time (day, week, month, year). It can also be used to calculate by Specialty, e.g. Cardio-Thoracic, Neurosurgery, Orthopedic, O&G, etc.

Brownfield Facility/Project

> A term used to describe an existing building, site location, or business that is experiencing a transfer of ownership e.g. an existing Hospital; or, another building that will be retrofitted or renovated from its current configuration into a Hospital or other type medical facility. Essentially it relates to a pre-existing facility, building, or on-going business entity.

Business Continuity Project/Management (BCP/M)

> Business Continuity Planning and Management is a subset of *Enterprise Risk Management (ERM)* with a specific focus on disruptive events that could affect access to the physical facilities, or disrupt the organizations ability to provide the basic services or workflow for a pre-determined period of time. The goal is to identify all potential threats, assess them and prepare a holistic, proactive, integrated set of plans to respond to a Disruptive Event. The ultimate objective is to protect People, Physical, and Intellectual Property to ensure continuity of their defined Critical Business Functions (CBFs).

Capacity Factor (CF)

> The optimal number of procedures, tests, images, cycles, and other services that can be performed within the defined time for which they will be operational. They will be assigned a realistic Efficiency Factor (EF), and the result will become the denominator when determining percentage of operation metric, with the actual number used as the numerator. Example. An MRI machine takes "on average" 40 minutes

to complete a scan cycle. It is made available and operates, 10 hours per day (600 minutes) with an EF of 85%. Maximum number of MRIs that can be performed with this profile is an average of 12.75 MRIs per day. This is the Capacity Factor. This can be scaled up from day to week, month, and annual numbers. Same concept can be used to calculate the optimal number of appointments in a Clinic, tests to be performed by lab, pharmacy prescriptions filled, etc.

CAPEX

Capital Expenditures. Money spent for acquisition of buildings, major renovations, and equipment with value over a determined amount, that will be reported on the Balance Sheet, with an amount expensed during the reporting period as an expense in providing services.

Chief Executive Officer (CEO)

The CEO is the most Senior Administrative staff in the Organization. They report to the Board of Directors/Trustees, and have overall responsibility for performance of the healthcare facility, e.g., Hospital, Specialty Centers etc. The CEO provides guidance and sets strategic direction based on Board expectations. Ultimately, all staff in the organization report to the CEO via his direct "C-Suite" reports. In Academic Medical Centers, the equivalent title may be "Facility name" Medical Director.

Chief Financial Officer (CFO)

Most senior Financial Individual in a large institution who is responsible for the overall financial performance and operation, insurance, legal compliance, purchasing/contracting function, and reports directly to the CEO.

The CFO is also responsible for the preparation of the annual Budget, and administration of the approved Budget including financial performance metrics and statistical reporting.

Chief Information Officer (CIO)

In a large facility or at Group level, the most senior Information Technology Professional who reports to the COO with a dotted line reporting to the CEO depending on the organization, responsible for implementation, operations, testing, and security of organization wide computer software programs/systems, computer related equipment, server farms, Data Centers, and internal and external interfaces.

Chairman Medical Board (CMB)

Appointed Senior Medical Staff reporting directly the CEO, and with a "dotted line" relationship to the Board, responsible for managing all the Clinical Specialties offered by the organization, ensuring compliance with required licensure of the facility and Specialists, as well as, clinical standards and ethics. The individual may also Chair or participate in various key clinical committees, such as Accreditation, Credentialing, Ethics, Standards, Drug and Therapeutic,

Chief Nursing Officer (CNO)

Most Senior of Nurses reporting to the CEO, who is responsible for management of all nursing staff, from ensuring proper assignment to wards, education, and applicable nursing standards and provision of support services to the Doctors and Specialists. Works closely with all the "Chiefs" in Senior Administration.

Chief Operating Officer (COO)

>Senior non-Clinical Administrative staff within the Hospital or facility and who is responsible for all Allied Health, Ancillary Services, Facility Management, Environmental, and Foods Services to support the Clinical functions being performed. Either COO or CMB will provide coverage should CEO during times of absence.

Chronic Care

>Chronic Care Refers to medical conditions requiring long term care either in a Hospital, Long-Term Healthcare facility, or even at home with support of a mobile medical Team. Chronic care patients can experience situation where Acute Care may be required for a period of time, and then revert back to their chronic status.

Costing - Unit

>In the healthcare context, it is the process of identifying all the resources (direct, indirect-direct, and general overheads) used to perform a procedure or provide a service, e.g., consultation, surgery, teaching. Discreet costs are assigned to each component and the total cost can then be used for transfer of cost to other department(s), used in "bundling" of services, and ultimately developing a unit price of a procedure or service for billing purposes.

Critical Business Function (CBF)

>Within the Healthcare community, Critical Business Functions are the specified services within the Hospital or Healthcare facilities which need to be maintained and protected from unplanned interrupted during a Disastrous

Event. Examples of specified services are, OR/OTs, ICUs, A&E/ERs, Dialysis Units and part of various service departments to support the specified services, and utilities such as electrical, water, medical gas supply, etc.

Direct Cost

The cost of any good or service that contributes to, and is readily ascribable to a product or service provided. Direct expense includes salaries and wages, employee benefits, professional fees, supplies, purchased services, and other direct expenses.

Direct-Indirect Cost

A Department's fixed and/or non-billable administrative and operating expenses such as Department Head, Secretary, Clerks and common internal supply expenses, license fees, repairs and maintenance, etc. These expenses are normally aggregated and allocated as overheads to the Direct costs associated with revenue generating billable products, procedures and services. There must be a metric to serve as a basis for the allocation, usually number of procedures, direct cost proportions, or time.

Duty of Care

In a Healthcare context, the concept of "duty of care" represents both a legal, and moral responsibility of providing services commensurate with the Clinician's training and skillsets. The services and care provided would be expected to be comparable to what professional peers with the same or similar qualifications. Consultant level Specialist would have a greater "duty of care" responsibility than a Medical Officer, General Practitioner, or junior level Specialist.

Consequently, the more senior individuals are "expected" to have greater knowledge, and they in turn must conduct sufficient tests and procedures to comfortably "rule out" any other potential underlying causes for a patient's symptoms or condition, failing which the Specialist may be guilty of not keeping their patient safe from harm.

The same principle applies to all other professionals within the Healthcare facilities. The higher the level of individual in the organizational hierarchy, the greater the responsibility they have to ensure compliance with all rules and regulations, within their respective areas of expertise and by their staff, including Senior Management and Administration.

EBITDA (Earnings Before Interest, Taxes, Depreciation and Amortization)

1. Total Operating Revenue less Total Operating Expenses equals **Earnings**
2. **I**nterest. Interest paid on Debt Servicing
3. **T**axes. Income Tax
4. **D**epreciation. Decline in value of the acquisition cost of a Capital Asset as it is consumed over its Useful Life
5. **A**mortization. Decline in value of an Intangible Asset as it is consumed over a Useful Life, e.g. software, brand name, patent value, R&D costs, etc.

Earnings before ITDA are a measure of the Companies/ Organizations operational financial performance over a stipulated period of time for which the Management Team is responsible and forms the basis for Financial Reporting. Whereas, ITDA are related to Board determined Financial Structure (Debt vs Equity), and Taxes which are a function of the Government regulations and rates, both of which are not under direct operational Management control.

Efficiency Factor (EF)

Efficiency Factor is an allowance for the fact there will always be "nonproductive time" throughout the day. While one may be scheduled to work for eight or ten hours per, one will be unable to provide services for 100% of the time. Time will be lost because patients/customers may be late, computer/printer or other piece of equipment breaks down, run out of supplies and need to replenish, you may need to obtain a drink, go to the toilette, stretch one's legs, mid-morning and mid-afternoon break, walk around and take a break from the computer screen, make a few personal telephone calls, conduct an errand, work slower due to feeling ill (emerging flu or handover). All these activities detract from the 100% time at work, so one's actual productive work time, Efficiency Factor, is normally between 70-95%. For budgeting and planning purposes, 80% is normally used.

Epiphany

In the healthcare setting, a sudden realization or insight that a particular outcome can be satisfied using an existing procedure, or piece of equipment by modifying the sequence of steps in a procedure or upgrading software of an existing piece of equipment to achieve operational expectations. Useful in both research settings and situations where new services or medical practices are being initiated.

24 Hr Emergency Clinic

May be freestanding, independent services (separate from the hospital setting) where individuals my go for treatment of medical conditions 24 hr a day, and managed by a Team of GP/Resident doctors with Specialists "on call" in necessary but not immediately available. They will normally perform a "triage" function, for purposes of isolating patients presenting with diseases and severity of injury for medical care. They typically have access to Lab, Imaging, and Pharmacy services, but may not be part of the Emergency Service Ambulance network.

Emergency Room (ER)

Refer to Accident and Emergency Service description above.

Enterprise Risk Management (ERM)

Structured approach to address different types of risk within an organization, with a view to Avoid, Prevent, Mitigate/Minimize, Transfer where possible, and Accept residual risk or conditions where probability and/or impact of the event is negligible, or the cost of the incremental coverage is too great for the benefit to be covered. Risk must be reviewed across the entire spectrum of services and responsibilities of the organisation. Effective management of ERM will result in lower insurance premiums. Refer to Risk Management. Hospital Organizational Risks can be categorized into the following Groupings or equivalent:

1. Clinical, e.g. Confidentiality, Consent, Negligence, Treatment, Ethics, etc.
2. Financial, e.g. Currency, Fraud, Funding, Collections, Investment, Internal Control, Exchange Rates, etc.
3. Legal, e.g. Shareholding Type, Ownership (Title), Libel/Slander, Intellectual Property
4. Technology, e.g. Medical Equipment, IT Systems (Hacking, Failures of H/W and S/W Redundancy) etc.
5. Operational, e.g. Facilities (BCP/M), Falls, Accidents/Incidents, Vehicles, Security shortfalls, etc.

6. Human Resources, e.g. Manpower, Worker Comp, Insurance, References
7. Strategic, e.g., Governance, Forward Planning, Risk Appetite, etc.

Full-Time Equivalent (FTE) Employee

Measurement of the number of personnel employed/engaged by a healthcare facility in terms of equivalent "Full Time" labour capability or requirement. To calculate the number of Full Time Equivalent employees, total all hours for which all employees are paid (whether worked or not) during the year/month and divide by:

Work Week (hrs)	Annual Non-Leap	Annual Leap	Month
40	2080	2088	173
42	2184	2192	182
44	2288	2296	191

Management uses the FTE concept for budgeting and as monitoring tool to measure performance, productivity measurement, workload, and staffing costs on a per employee basis. This can be reported by Individual, Department, Division, or Hospital Level, as well as by specialty; eg Medical, Nursing, Paraprofessional, Facility Support, Administrative (clerical), Executive. Normally used by HR, Finance, and Management to manage/monitor staffing levels relative to workload. The concept should also be used for measuring and quantifying "outsourced" services and "overtime hours" added to "core payroll" staff to obtain the complete complement of staff utilized by the organization. This allows for "like for like" comparisons between facilities.

General Overhead Costs

>Allocated share of organization wide administrative department expenses to all departments based on an acceptable statistic or metric. Examples: Executive Management (CEO, CFO, COO, CNO, CMB, etc.) Department costs allocated by FTEs, Human Resource Costs allocated based on the number of FTE in each Department, Utilities and Environmental Services etc. based on square footage. Amounts vary depending on the number of Revenue Generating Departments within the organization.

Greenfield Facility/Project

>A term used to convey construction of a new facility, normally a building on an undeveloped or cleared plot of land that has been zoned for the intended purposes, and built based on a set of architectural drawings. The term may also be used to also convey start-up of a new Project

Headcount

>The physical body count of all employees working for an organisation, both as full and part time employees. This number may differ from Full Time Equivalents (FTE). When all employees are working full time, then Headcount will equal Full Time Equivalent. Headcount management is useful for work schedule planning, or provision of services during peak service times. It is also critical for reporting, and insurance purposes.

Eg	Working	Headcount	FTE
	1 Staff, full time	1	1.0
	2 Staff, ½ Time	2	1.0
	4 Staff, ¼ Time	4	1.0
	1 Staff, ½ Time	1	0.5

Hand-Foot-Mouth Disease (HFMD)

A common contagious viral infection caused by a strain of Coxsackie disease amongst infants and children. It is often spread at Child Nurseries, Day Care Centers, Pre-school, Kindergartens, and through lower primary school grades. Symptoms identified with the disease are blisters on the hands, feet, with painful mouth and throat sores which typically last for about 7-10 days.

Hospital

A Ministry Licensed, and Certified establishment providing observation, diagnostic, and treatment services to patients by an organised group of medical and professional staff, normally located in a permanent physical structure. Hospital facilities typically include a range of inpatient beds, eg, General (Lying in), HD (Progressive), and Intensive Care Units (ICU), medical services, continuous nursing services, Ancillary Support /Allied Health Services (Pharmacy, Laboratory, Imaging, Rehab, etc.), Operational Support (Bio-Med Engineering Dietary, Housekeeping, Facility Maintenance, Laundry, Food Service Catering, etc.), to support the medical/nursing staff of the facility. Hospitals may be classified and General Acute, Secondary, Tertiary, or Quaternary, levels. There are also Rehabilitation, Specialty, and Community Hospitals.

Hospital-Based Physician/Doctor

A Specialist/Doctor who is an employee of the hospital and spends the majority of their practice time within one or more affiliated hospitals instead of being in an independent provider, in a private office setting, with admission privileges. A Hospital-based Specialist/Doctor usually has a financial arrangement with the hospital, i.e. being an employee (salary and/or percentage of fees generated, and/or bonus thresholds). Such specialist/doctors usually include Medical Directors or Medical education, Pathologists, Anaesthesiologist and Radiologists, as well as the Medical Officers or Resident Physicians who staff the Emergency Room, 24 Hr Clinics, and provide back-up medical support to the wards.

Independent Doctor/Specialist

A Doctor/Specialist who maintains an independent medical practice treating patients within their office who are not in the direct employ of the hospital. They will also be granted "admitting privileges" to one or more hospitals in the surrounding area with access to medical support services (inpatient beds, Operating Theatres, treatment facilities, diagnostic equipment, laboratory rehabilitation services, etc.). The Hospital and the Doctor will bill the patient independently (however, in many instances the Hospital will facilitate by including the Specialists Charges in the patient's bill and collect on their behalf, remitting the collections to the Specialist upon collection).

Information Technology

Term used to capture infrastructure implementation to support of computers, printers, servers, software, and related peripheral devices for collection, processing, storage (local or cloud), report writing, sharing of information to eligible, approved individuals or entities.

Intensive Care (Medical, Surgical, Cardiac, Neonatal, Neuro, etc.)

Services provided in an inpatient care unit to patients who require extraordinary observation and care on a concentrated, exhaustive and continuous basis. Intensive care patients normally receive between 18-24 hours (1:1) of direct "hands-on" care, treatment, or constant monitoring per day. Because of the high ratio of Doctors and Nurses time involved in service provision, this is the most expensive level of care offered by a Hospital.

Intensity Factor

A mathematical relationship between an independent occurrence and the subsequent activity generated as a result of the event. An example - one patient admission will result in an average of two radiological procedures being performed; six Labs test ordered; four prescriptions provided; three meals being provided per day, etc. A technique that ensures all the services are properly correlated with changes in workload, to ensure proper service planning and delivery. Once the data is collected, it can be used for both budgetary, and daily scheduling, eg nurses to different specialties.

Medical Director (MD)

An alternate title to CEO for the most senior individual responsible for the Healthcare facility. Used most frequently in an Academic Healthcare environment.

OPEX

Operating Expenditures. Sum of all the direct normal line items expenses listed on an Income Statement (P/L), e.g. Salaries/Wages/Benefits, Fees, Supplies, Consumables, COGS, Utilities, etc.

PEST Analysis

A structured analytical tool used by organizations to identify and address external elements that can impact a current business situation. The abbreviation stands for: Political, Environmental, Socio-Cultural, and Technological. List all relevant conditions under each of the four category definitions, analyze them, and determine what actions to take to improve the organizations current situation or to consider before embarking on a new project. PEST analysis can be used to supplement a SWOT analysis, as the focus is different.

Policy & Procedure (P&P) Manuals

Collection of Organizational and Departmental documents addressing policies, principles, and concepts. They may include an organisation chart; staffing requirements; operational, and service quality standards; procedures on how to perform various treatments; guidelines and checklist; chart of accounts with relevant definitions; standard units of measure; performance standards which establishes a foundation for consistency in performance and delivery of services, uniform reporting, and data collection. A proper set of P&P will normally provide direction and guidelines for about 95% of all routine activities in an organisation. Having proper P&Ps in place are critical for MOH Licensing initial application and subsequent renewal, as well as various

Accreditation bodies, eg JCI, ISO, SQA/C, People Developer, etc. Also known as *Standard Operating Procedures (SOPs)* with a slightly different template.

Pro-Forma

A financial model for either the Profit/Loss Income Statement (P/L) or Balance Sheet (BS) and represents a future projection for Budget Projections of current operations, or planning for a new project. It starts with a template using current P/L lines (high level or detailed) and then make a list of "assumptions" for Workload (volume), Revenue (price changes +/-), Expense (cost changes +/-), inflation, and interest rates. Most Pro-Formas will start with the current year, then expanded for the next 1, 3, 5, 10, 20 years, with assumptions for each year, and also including major capital infusion (renovations, equipment, new building), new programs or projects and their financial impacts. Pro-Formas should be transparent in design and build up.

SARS

Abbreviation stands for Severe Acute Respiratory Syndrome. It is a contagious respiratory disease (pneumonia) caused by a virus, and emerged from China in 2002/03 and spread internationally.

Standard Operating Procedure (SOP)

Refer to Policy & Procedure above.

SWOT Analysis

A structured analytical tool used by organizations to identify and address a current or potential business environment.

The abbreviation stands for: Strengths, Weaknesses, Opportunities and Threats. List all relevant descriptions under each of the four category definitions, analyze them, and determine what actions to take to improve the organizations current situation or to consider before embarking on a new project.

Workload Optimization

Based on the Capacity Factor (CF) of any piece of equipment, available workspace space or manpower, it is the practice of generating sufficient workload to raise the use of the resource to 95-98% utilization. To achieve such utilization is may be necessary to introduce new uses or users of equipment, e.g. actively seek out contracts with GPs or Specialists to refer their patients to the Hospital or Center to meet their imaging requirements, provide labs services, or for excess space, explore renting or leasing out "vacant" space pending internal growth and taking back the space. Refer to Capacity Factor definition and calculation.

SUBJECT INDEX

		Page
Business Office		
I:9	Final Reminder Notification	18
I:11	Medi-Series, Understanding (Singapore)	22
II:46	Pricing – To Local Market Rates	126
Clinical		
III:15	Clinical Discipline Balance	193
III:40	Delays, Dr/Specialist Waiting Time	231
II:40	Doctor "Buy In"	113
II:20	Doctors Must Drive Clinical Initiatives	70
II:35	Doctor's/Specialist's Experience Epiphany	101
II:51	Duty of Care Responsibility	136
II:37	Leaving for Private Practice, Reasons	106
II:47	Medical Staff Growth, Timing	128
II:18	Meetings with Doctors/Specialists	67
II:38	Skills and EQ, Combinations	110
II:62	Specialist Recruitment	163
II:52	Specialist Referral Network, Development	139
I:13	Value of Doctor Assessment	26
II:49	Value Patients as a Resource	133

Corporate Communications

II:50	Cost – Manpower	....	134
II:56	Cost of Care – Services	....	149
II:57	Cost of Care – Users	....	153
II:55	Cost of Drugs - Hospital	....	146
III:30	Managing AV Equipment	....	214
II:36	Public and Private Practices, Differences	....	103

Customer Relations

II:1	"Frequent Flyer" Offers	....	37
I:7	Hope!	....	13
I:10	Number of Shortcomings	....	19
I:6	See You Soon!	....	12
I:3	Smile!	....	6

Common Sense

IV:10	Battery Failure	....	286
IV:13	Have a GREAT Day	....	289
IV:8	Saving Best for Last?	....	284
IV:9	Telephone Interruptions	....	285
IV:7	Too Good to be True!	....	283
IV:11	Too Much Work	....	286

Finance

III:45	Feasibility Study	....	241
III:44	FX Rates – Unfavourable	....	241
I:12	Identify Root Causes	....	23
III:24	Insurance Lapses	....	205
II:23	Manpower Reduction Management	....	75
III:46	Pricing Related Decisions	....	244
II:43	Remember the "3R"s	....	118
II:30	Validate Data	....	89

Human Resources

III:56	Avoid Appraisal Delay	....	262
IV:4	Books Purchased vs Free	....	280
II:59	Business "Partner" Recognition	....	159
III:57	Chronological Recording	....	263
III:54	Climbing Career Ladder	....	259
II:39	Clinical vs Administrative Skills	....	112
II:32	Golden Handcuff, Use of	....	94
IV:5	Grass is Burnt	....	281
III:51	Integrity, Motivation, Ethics	....	254
III:28	Loyalty	....	211
III:9	No Second Chances	....	182
II:61	Physically Challenged Individuals, Use	....	162
III:55	Record of all Personnel, Maintain	....	260
III:58	Retired Staff, Maintain Contact	....	265
III:52	Sabotaging "Peers"	....	256
II:60	Verifying Surgical Teamwork	....	160
IV:12	Working Beyond Retirement Age	....	288

IT

III:22	Computer "Hangs"	....	203
III:10	Look to the Computer	....	184
II:19	Understand Linkages	....	69

Operations - General

III:23	Administrators are "Janitors"	....	204
III:60	Administrative Staff Perspective	....	272
III:14	Audit Recommendations	....	191
III:13	Audit Report Card	....	190
III:12	Audit Sample Selection	....	187
III:11	Auditor Training	....	186
I:14	Documentation Missing, Not Done	....	28
III:42	Document Discrepancies	....	238
IV:2	Dumb vs Smart	....	278

III:35	Effective Signage Testing	......	221
II:15	Employment – Healthcare Professional	......	62
III:37	Idea Development	......	225
III:53	Knowing Right from Wrong	......	257
II:12	Life in a "Chief" Role	......	56
II:31	Professional Distancing	......	92
II:58	Service Quality	......	156
III:4	Sign It, Own It	......	174
IV:6	Tidy Work Area	......	282
III:38	Transparency	......	226
III:43	Translation Accuracy	......	240
III:47	Staff Productivity	......	247
IV:3	Updated CV	......	279

Operational Management

II:24	Ask WHY	......	79
III:36	Avoid "Blind-Siding"	......	223
III:16	Brief The Chairman	......	194
III:31	Bring Me a Problem, and Solutions	......	216
III:27	Capitalize on Individual Strength	......	210
III:20	Catching vs Chasing	......	201
II:42	Clinical Politics	......	116
III:5	Decision Implications	......	176
III:32	Eclectic Style Management, Use of	......	218
II:5	"Friends" with Competition	......	44
IV:1	Friends like You, Need No Enemies	......	277
II:21	Initiative Success, F(x) of Timing	......	71
III:25	Late for Work/Meeting	......	206
II:45	Living Within Budget, Trade-offs	......	124
III:39	Management of Expired Drugs	......	228
III:50	Minutes per Slide	......	253
III:2	More Complex the Question, Less Time	......	170
II:16	Negotiating Contract Terms	......	64
III:29	Never Free, Time Precious	......	213

II:44	"Non-Profit" Status, Understanding	....	122
III:6	Observe Procedures, Learn	....	177
III:41	Predecessor Comments	....	236
III:49	Presentations and Learning	....	252
III:7	Same Thing, Only Different	....	179
III:3	Share Background	....	172
III:19	Supporters	....	200
III:33	Taking Minutes/Notes	....	219
III:21	Taxies "Drying Up"	....	202
II:8	Unique Solutions, Finding	....	49
II:25	Use of Consultants, Reasons Why	....	80
I:15	Use of ER/A&E, Proper	....	29
II:3	Walk the Talk	....	39
III:18	When Most Crisis Occur	....	198

Organization

II:33	BCP (Business Continuity Planning)	....	96
II:2	Higher Level Re-Organization	....	38
II:26	Hiring Previously Engaged Consultants	....	82
III:8	Organization Change Cycle Repeat	....	180
II:27	Ownership of Department, Organization	....	84
II:29	Ownership of Financial Data	....	87
II:13	P&P Usefulness	....	58
II:28	Stewardship Duties, Responsibilities	....	86
III:34	Successors Will Make Changes	....	220

Professionalism

III:17	Being a Mentor	....	196
I:1	Demonstrate Good Hygiene	....	3
I:2	Dressing and Acting as Professionals	....	4

Planning

II:7	Build/Construct Facilities for Long Term	....	47
II:6	Building Hospitals	....	46

II:4	Hospital Planning and Closets	....	42
II:54	Patient Areas Functional and Zoned	....	145

Purchasing

III:48	Life Cycle Analysis	....	249
II:9	Reputable Sources, Using	....	50
II:34	Vendor Sponsored Trips, Caution	....	99

Strategic

III:59	Adoption of Accreditation Standards	....	267
II:53	Good Clinical Outcomes	....	142
III:26	Great Number Two	....	208
II:10	Healthcare always Relevant	....	52
II:11	Healthcare Fascinating Industry	....	55
II:17	Holistic Perspective	....	65
II:48	Land for Equity Ownership, Donation	....	130
II:41	Offering Clinical Back-up Services	....	114
II:22	Sensitive Solutions	....	73
II:14	Strategic Partners, Extended Staff	....	60

Writing

I:16	Delay Response to Negative Feedback	....	32
I:8	Letter Writing, First Response	....	16
I:4	Non-Attackable Lead In, Use of	....	7
I:5	Use of Negative Words, Avoid	....	10
III:1	Write from Reader's Perspective	....	169

www.ingramcontent.com/pod-product-compliance
Lightning Source LLC
Chambersburg PA
CBHW020726180526
45163CB00001B/128